Clinicians' Guides to Radionuclide Hybrid Imaging

PET/CT

Series editors

Jamshed B. Bomanji
London, UK

Gopinath Gnanasegaran
London, UK

Stefano Fanti
Bologna, Italy

Homer A. Macapinlac
Houston, Texas, USA

More information about this series at http://www.springer.com/series/13803

Sue Chua
Editor

PET/CT in Radiotherapy Planning

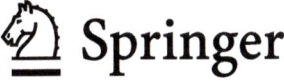

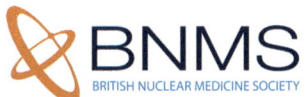

Editor
Sue Chua
Department of Nuclear Medicine and PET
Royal Marsden NHS Foundation Trust
Sutton
Surrey
United Kingdom

ISSN 2367-2439   ISSN 2367-2447 (electronic)
Clinicians' Guides to Radionuclide Hybrid Imaging - PET/CT
ISBN 978-3-319-54743-5   ISBN 978-3-319-54744-2 (eBook)
DOI 10.1007/978-3-319-54744-2

Library of Congress Control Number: 2017942962

© Springer International Publishing Switzerland 2017
This work is subject to copyright. All rights are reserved by the Publisher, whether the whole or part of the material is concerned, specifically the rights of translation, reprinting, reuse of illustrations, recitation, broadcasting, reproduction on microfilms or in any other physical way, and transmission or information storage and retrieval, electronic adaptation, computer software, or by similar or dissimilar methodology now known or hereafter developed.
The use of general descriptive names, registered names, trademarks, service marks, etc. in this publication does not imply, even in the absence of a specific statement, that such names are exempt from the relevant protective laws and regulations and therefore free for general use.
The publisher, the authors and the editors are safe to assume that the advice and information in this book are believed to be true and accurate at the date of publication. Neither the publisher nor the authors or the editors give a warranty, express or implied, with respect to the material contained herein or for any errors or omissions that may have been made. The publisher remains neutral with regard to jurisdictional claims in published maps and institutional affiliations.

Printed on acid-free paper

This Springer imprint is published by Springer Nature
The registered company is Springer International Publishing AG
The registered company address is: Gewerbestrasse 11, 6330 Cham, Switzerland

PET/CT series is dedicated to Prof Ignac Fogelman, Dr Muriel Buxton-Thomas and Prof Ajit K Padhy

Foreword

Clear and concise clinical indications for PET/CT in the management of the oncology patient are presented in this series of 15 separate booklets.

The impact on better staging, tailored management and specific treatment of the patient with cancer has been achieved with the advent of this multimodality imaging technology. Early and accurate diagnosis will always pay, and clear information can be gathered with PET/CT on treatment responses. Prognostic information is gathered and can further guide additional therapeutic options.

It is a fortunate coincidence that PET/CT was able to derive great benefit from radionuclide-labelled probes, which deliver good and often excellent target to non-target signals. Whilst labelled glucose remains the cornerstone for the clinical benefit achieved, a number of recent probes are definitely adding benefit. PET/CT is hence an evolving technology, extending its applications and indications. Significant advances in the instrumentation and data processing available have also contributed to this technology, which delivers high throughput and a wealth of data, with good patient tolerance and indeed patient and public acceptance. As an example, the role of PET/CT in the evaluation of cardiac disease is also covered, with emphasis on labelled rubidium and labelled glucose studies.

The novel probes of labelled choline; labelled peptides, such as DOTATATE; and, most recently, labelled PSMA (prostate-specific membrane antigen) have gained rapid clinical utility and acceptance, as significant PET/CT tools for the management of neuroendocrine disease and prostate cancer patients, notwithstanding all the advances achieved with other imaging modalities, such as MRI. Hence, a chapter reviewing novel PET tracers forms part of this series.

The oncological community has recognised the value of PET/CT and has delivered advanced diagnostic criteria for some of the most important indications for PET/CT. This includes the recent Deauville criteria for the classification of PET/CT patients with lymphoma—similar criteria are expected to develop for other malignancies, such as head and neck cancer, melanoma and pelvic malignancies. For completion, a separate section covers the role of PET/CT in radiotherapy planning, discussing the indications for planning biological tumour volumes in relevant cancers.

These booklets offer simple, rapid and concise guidelines on the utility of PET/CT in a range of oncological indications. They also deliver a rapid aide-memoire on the merits and appropriate indications for PET/CT in oncology.

London, UK											Peter J. Ell, FMedSci, DR HC, AΩA

Preface

Hybrid imaging with PET/CT and SPECT/CT combines the best of function and structure to provide accurate localisation, characterisation and diagnosis. There are extensive literature and evidence to support PET/CT, which have made significant impact in oncological imaging and management of patients with cancer. The evidence in favour of SPECT/CT especially in orthopaedic indications is evolving and increasing.

The *Clinicians' Guide to Radionuclide Hybrid Imaging* pocketbook series is specifically aimed at our referring clinicians, nuclear medicine/radiology doctors, radiographers/technologists and nurses who are routinely working in nuclear medicine and participate in multidisciplinary meetings. This series is the joint work of many friends and professionals from different nations who share a common dream and vision towards promoting and supporting nuclear medicine as a useful and important imaging speciality.

We want to thank all those people who have contributed to this work as advisors, authors and reviewers, without whom the book would not have been possible. We want to thank our members from the BNMS (British Nuclear Medicine Society, UK) for their encouragement and support, and we are extremely grateful to Dr Brian Nielly, Charlotte Weston, the BNMS Education Committee and the BNMS council members for their enthusiasm and trust.

Finally, we wish to extend particular gratitude to the industry for their continuous supports towards education and training.

London, UK
                                                                                              Jamshed Bomanji
                                                                                            Gopinath Gnanasegaran

Acknowledgements

The series coordinators and editors would like to express their sincere gratitude to the members of the British Nuclear Medicine Society, patients, teachers, colleagues, students, industry and BNMS Education Committee members, for their continued support and inspiration:

Andy Bradley
Brent Drake
Francis Sundram
James Ballinger
Parthiban Arumugam
Rizwan Syed
Sai Han
Vineet Prakash

Contents

Part I Radiotherapy Planning in Oncology: Science and Practice

1 **Introduction**... 3
Lucy Fowkes and Kate Newbold

Part II PET/CT in Radiotherapy Planning - Technical and Practical Aspects

2 **Instrumentation**... 13
Alex Dunlop

3 **Patient Preparation**... 17
Clare Ockwell and Shirley Summers

4 **Data Acquisition, Reconstruction and Transfer**................. 23
David Towey and Laurence Hill

5 **Sources of Artefacts: Consequences and Solutions**.............. 29
Alison Tree and Maria Hawkins

6 **Advantages and Limitations**.................................. 33
Shaista Hafeez and Robert Huddart

7 **4D PET/CT Respiratory Gated Acquisition Techniques**............ 39
Iain Murray

Part III PET/CT in Radiotherapy Planning - Current Evidence and Applications

8 **Lung Cancer**.. 45
Angus O'Connor and Helen M. Betts

9 **Head and Neck Cancers**...................................... 51
Liam Welsh and Kate Newbold

10 **GI Malignancy**... 57
Irene Chong and Diana Tait

11	**Prostate Cancer**...	63
	Daniel R. Henderson and Nicholas van As	
12	**Gynaecological Cancers**.....................................	67
	Susan Lalondrelle	
13	**Paediatric Tumours**...	73
	Lucy Fowkes and Sue Chua	

Index... 77

Contributors

Nicholas van As The Royal Marsden NHS Foundation Trust, London, UK

Helen M. Betts Department of Medical Physics and Clinical Engineering, Nottingham University Hospitals NHS Trust, Nottingham, UK

Irene Chong The Royal Marsden NHS Foundation Trust, London, UK

Sue Chua Department of Nuclear Medicine and PET, Royal Marsden NHS Foundation Trust, Sutton, Surrey, UK

Alex Dunlop Department of Radiotherapy, The Royal Marsden NHS Foundation Trust, London, UK

Lucy Fowkes The Royal Marsden NHS Foundation Trust, London, UK

Shaista Hafeez The Royal Marsden NHS Foundation Trust and The Institute of Cancer Research, Sutton, Surrey, UK
The Royal Marsden NHS Foundation Trust, London, UK

Maria Hawkins CRUK MRC Oxford Institute for Radiation Oncology, Gray Laboratories, University of Oxford, Oxford, UK

Daniel R. Henderson The Royal Marsden NHS Foundation Trust, London, UK

Laurence Hill Radiological Sciences Unit, Imperial College Healthcare NHS Trust, London, UK

Robert Huddart The Institute of Cancer Research, The Royal Marsden NHS Foundation Trust, London, UK

Susan Lalondrelle The Royal Marsden NHS Foundation Trust, London, UK

Iain Murray The Royal Marsden NHS Foundation Trust, London, UK

Kate Newbold The Royal Marsden NHS Foundation Trust, London, UK

Angus O'Connor Department of Radiology, Nottingham University Hospitals NHS Trust, Hucknall Road, Nottingham, UK

Clara Ockwell Department of Radiotherapy, The Royal Marsden NHS Foundation Trust, London, UK

Shirley Summers Nuclear Medicine and PET Department, The Royal Marsden NHS Foundation Trust, London, UK

Diana Tait The Royal Marsden NHS Foundation Trust, London, UK

David Towey Radiological Sciences Unit, Imperial College Healthcare NHS Trust, London, UK

Alison Tree Royal Marsden NHS Foundation Trust, London, UK

Liam Welsh The Royal Marsden NHS Foundation Trust, London, UK

Part I

Radiotherapy Planning in Oncology: Science and Practice

Introduction

Lucy Fowkes and Kate Newbold

Contents

1.1 Introduction 3
1.2 EBRT Planning Process 4
1.3 Role of PET/CT in RT Planning 4
1.4 PET-MRI 7
References 9

1.1 Introduction

Worldwide, cancer is a major public health issue and accurate diagnosis, staging and follow-up is essential for optimal management. PET/CT imaging has a significant role in the staging of disease and assessment of treatment response.

External beam radiotherapy (EBRT) is used in the treatment of approximately 40% of cancer patients [1]. The function of EBRT is to destroy or control the growth of malignant cells, and the EBRT planning process aims to achieve maximal therapeutic effect whilst keeping levels of toxicity to a minimum.

L. Fowkes
Radiology & Radionuclide Radiology, The Royal Marsden NHS Foundation Trust, London, UK

K. Newbold (✉)
Head & Neck and Thyroid Unit, The Royal Marsden NHS Foundation Trust and Institute of Cancer Research, London, UK

Clinical Oncology, The Royal Marsden NHS Foundation Trust, London, UK
e-mail: kate.newbold@rmh.nhs.uk

The planning of EBRT is heavily reliant upon imaging modalities to (a) accurately identify the radiation target volumes in order to avoid geographical misses of disease sites and (b) to confidently define and spare normal organs at risk of damage from radiation. CT also provides electron density data via the Hounsfield units required for dosimetric calculation in EBRT planning. Standardly EBRT planning has been performed using anatomical imaging such as CT or MRI; however the combination of functional and anatomical imaging in PET/CT also provides information regarding tumour biology. Such data serves to inform treatment, particularly in the case of EBRT, and also provides a more sensitive measurement of treatment response, than conventional imaging, in a number of tumours [2].

1.2 EBRT Planning Process

Imaging data is integral to the RT treatment planning system, and a number of target volumes (Fig. 1.1) are defined in accordance with the recommendations of the International Commission of Radiation Units and Measurements. Organs at risk (OAR) are defined in order that dose is maintained within tolerable limits to these structures minimising long-term toxicity [3].

1.3 Role of PET/CT in RT Planning

The PET component of PET/CT utilises various tracers to provide information regarding the molecular behaviour of a tumour, whether this be its metabolism, rate of apoptosis, level of hypoxia, proliferation or particular gene expression.

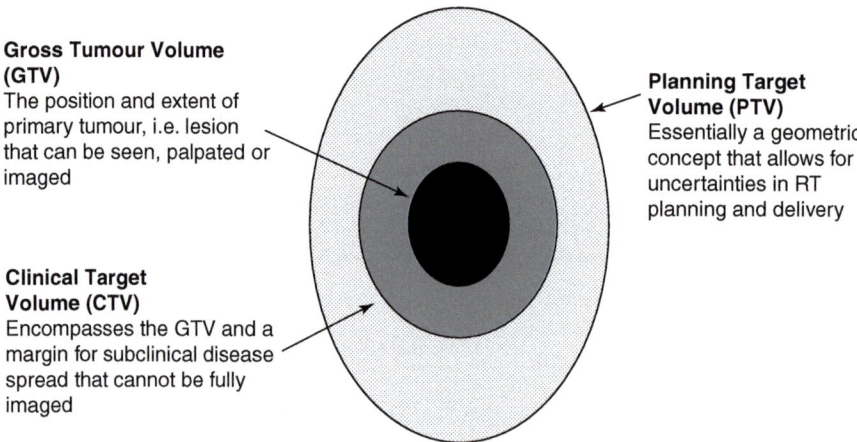

Fig. 1.1 Target volumes in radiotherapy

The co-registration of this biological information with anatomical imaging can provide invaluable information for the radiation oncologist when planning radiation delivery to the tumour. In addition to superior localization of disease through improved staging, dose escalation to potentially radioresistant subvolumes or change in treatment modality if lack of response to initial treatment may be permitted.

Functional changes often precede morphological ones, for example, changes in tumour glucose metabolism manifest as altered ^{18}F-FDG accumulation and predict changes in tumour volume [4] that cannot yet be detected upon conventional imaging. Differentiating viable tumour from adjacent structures is sometimes difficult with morphological imaging, particularly if the anatomy has been altered by previous treatment. Specific examples include regions of complex anatomy, for instance, in the head and neck region where tumour has been resected and subsequent reconstruction with muscle or bone grafts has occurred, or distinguishing between atelectasis and lung cancer. In such situations gross tumour volume (GTV) (Fig. 1.1) definition using PET/CT may be more accurate than CT alone [5] permitting reduced margins of uncertainty in target definition and hence potentially lessening normal tissue toxicity.

Data provided by PET may also modify the clinical target volume (CTV), for example, with the inclusion of metastatic lymph nodes not detected upon conventional morphological imaging. This was effectively demonstrated by a study of the impact of ^{18}F-FDG PET/CT upon the staging of solid tumours in a cohort of 260 patients in which nodal status was correctly identified by PET/CT in 92% of patients compared to 76% by CT. Fifteen percent of the patients studied had their treatment regimens altered following PET/CT [6].

Information provided by a PET study can be used to derive functional subvolumes (or biological target volumes (BTV)) within the CT/anatomical GTV. This concept lends itself to "dose painting" [7], with targeting of increased radiation dose to the most functionally active regions of the tumour or to overcome possible radioresistance in order to achieve better treatment outcomes. This may be performed by application of a homogeneous radiation dose to a PET defined BTV (dose painting by contours) or a heterogeneous radiation dose titrated in accordance with spatial variations in functional activity at a voxel level within a tumour volume (dose painting by numbers) [7].

PET data has been used to employ these methods in head and neck, lung and rectal [7] cancers with promising results.

Although FDG-PET/CT is used routinely within the clinic, other tracers and their use in radiotherapy planning remain within the research arena (Table 1.1). Further study is required as these agents often possess inherent biological uncertainties that may affect image interpretation particularly in relation to the spatial and temporal stability of PET imaging parameters during the course of treatment.

At present there is no consensus upon to how best delineate GTV upon PET. At its simplest, target volumes are defined by visual assessment, and this remains the most frequently used method, although this is subject to significant interobserver variability [16].

Table 1.1 Examples of PET tracers used in oncology

Cellular pathway utilised	Molecular basis	Tracer examples	Use
Amino acid transport and protein synthesis	Increased rates of amino acid transport [8]	*18F-FET*[a]	Brain tumour diagnosis, target volume delineation and follow-up
		18F-DOPA	Diagnosis and staging of neuroendocrine and brain tumours
		11C-MET	To define extent of glioma and detect its recurrence post-treatment
Glucose metabolism	Increased rates of glycolysis overexpression of GLUT-1 and three receptors, and increased levels mitochondrial hexokinase [9] in malignant cells	18F-FDG	Tumour detection and staging. Target volume delineation of multiple malignancies. Monitoring of treatment response
Apoptosis	Tumour apoptosis is often associated with a response to treatment. Small molecular probes detect activation of specific enzymes (specifically caspases), loss of mitochondrial membrane electrochemical potential or alterations in cell membrane composition (termed the apoptotic cellular imprint) occurring during apoptosis [10]	*18F-ML10*[a]	Potential role in the evaluation of therapeutic response to treatment [11]
Proliferation	Increased levels thymidine kinase in malignant/proliferating cells	*18F-FLT*[a]	Tumour detection, staging, restaging and assessment of treatment response [12]
Hypoxia	Tracers very permeable to cell membrane: at normal oxygen levels tracer diffuses in and out of cell, but in the presence of hypoxia intracellular nitroreductases alter its chemical structure and it becomes trapped within the cell. Tumour hypoxia indicates resistance to RT and tumour progression [13]	*18F-MISO*[a] *18F-FAZA*[a] *64Cu-ATSM*[a]	Identification of hypoxic regions within a variety of tumours potentially facilitating biological target volume definition and image-guided adaptive RT

Table 1.1 (continued)

Cellular pathway utilised	Molecular basis	Tracer examples	Use
Lipid metabolism	Neoplastic cells exhibit increased levels of phosphorylcholine	^{11}C-choline	Staging and detection of distant relapses in prostate cancer
		^{11}C-acetate	Detection of tumours for which FDG is ineffective, e.g. well-differentiated lung adenocarcinomas and HCC [14]
Angiogenesis	Targets integrin expressed by endothelial cells during vessel formation	^{18}F-$galacto$-RGD^a ^{18}F-$fluciclatide^a$	Possible predictive and prognostic biomarker
Somatostatin receptor	Receptors overexpressed in a number of tumours	^{68}Ga-DOTATOC ^{68}Ga-DOTATATE	Staging, follow-up, determine somatostatin receptor status for possible radioisotope therapy and assess treatment response primarily in neuroendocrine tumours [15]

[a]Denotes tracers under investigation
Where ^{11}C-MET ^{11}C-methionine, ^{18}F-FET ^{18}F-fluoroethyltyrosine, ^{18}F-$DOPA$ ^{18}F-fluorodopa, ^{18}F-FDG ^{18}F-fluorodeoxyglucose, ^{18}F-FLT 3′-deoxy-3′-^{18}F-fluorothymidine, ^{18}F-$ML10$ ^{18}F-2(5-fluoropentyl)-2-methylmalonic acid, ^{18}F-$MISO$ ^{8}F-fluoromisonidazole, ^{18}F-$FAZA$ ^{18}F-fluoroazomycin arabinoside, ^{64}Cu-$ATSM$ ^{64}Cu-diacetyl-bis(N4-methylthiosemicarbazone)

In response several automated semi-quantitative methods have been developed [17]. These include absolute maximum standardised uptake value (SUVmax) measurements, for example, for ^{18}F-FDG PET a SUVmax of 2.5 has been suggested as a threshold for GTV delineation. Percentages of SUVmax (often 40%) have also been used to define GTV. Other approaches including contrast-orientated, gradient-based, iterative and fuzzy clustering methods, along with source-to-background algorithms [17], have been explored. The gradient-based [18] and contrast orientation methods have proven promising; with the latter recommended for use in multicentre trials due to its high feasibility and repeatability [19].

1.4 PET-MRI

Hybrid PET-MRI systems allow multiple biological parameters and anatomical images of high spatial resolution to be obtained in a single acquisition. MR functional imaging techniques, such as diffusion-weighted (DWI) and dynamic contrast-enhanced (DCE) imaging, enable various pathophysiological tumour characteristics, including metabolism, perfusion, vascularisation and hypoxia, to be assessed simultaneously. This data can then be used to more precisely delineate tumours and so facilitate treatment planning, including dose painting for RT. Another potential advantage of PET-MRI is in monitoring treatment response and disease follow-up.

At present technical challenges relating to patient positioning, potential geometrical distortion of MR images and the effect of MR attenuation correction upon PET quantification need to be overcome before it is more widely practiced [20].

Conclusion

The biological information provided by PET helps to more accurately delineate disease extent in several tumour sites. This facilitates the implementation of more definitive cancer treatment and reduces radiation injury to surrounding tissues. Advances in RT precision delivery, development of novel PET tracers and continuing expansion of PET-MRI will further refine the RT planning process.

Key Points

- EBRT planning process aims to achieve maximal therapeutic effect whilst keeping levels of toxicity to a minimum.
- Conventional EBRT planning is performed using anatomical imaging such as CT or MRI.
- Combination of functional and anatomical imaging in PET/CT may provide information regarding tumour biology.
- The co-registration of this biological information with anatomical imaging can provide invaluable information for the radiation oncologist when planning radiation delivery to the tumour.
- Differentiating viable tumour from adjacent structures is sometimes difficult with morphological imaging, particularly if the anatomy has been altered by previous treatment. In such situations GTV definition using PET/CT may be more accurate than CT alone.
- Data provided by PET may also modify the CTV and functional subvolumes (or biological target volumes (BTV) within the CT/anatomical GTV.
- Currently, there is no consensus upon to how best delineate GTV upon PET.
- Hybrid PET-MRI systems allow multiple biological parameters and anatomical images of high spatial resolution to be obtained in a single acquisition.
- At present technical challenges relating to patient positioning, potential geometrical distortion of MR images and the effect of MR attenuation correction upon PET quantification need to be overcome before it is more widely practiced.

References

1. Cancer Research UK. What radiotherapy is. 2014. http://www.cancerresearchuk.org/about-cancer/cancers-in-general/treatment/radiotherapy/about/what-radiotherapy-is. Accessed 9 Jan 2015.
2. Wahl RL, Jacene H, Kasamon Y, Lodge MA. From RECIST to PERCIST: evolving considerations for PET response criteria in solid tumors. J Nucl Med. 2009;50(Suppl 1):122S–50S.
3. Berthelsen AK, Dobbs J, Kjellen E, et al. What's new in target volume definition for radiologists in ICRU report 71? How can the ICRU volume definitions be integrated in clinical practice? Cancer Imaging. 2007;7:104–16.
4. Ben-Haim S, Ell P. ^{18}F-FDG PET and PET/CT in the evaluation of cancer treatment response. J Nucl Med. 2009;50(1):88–99.
5. Nestle U, Walter K, Schmidt S, et al. 18F-deoxyglucose positron emission tomography (FDG-PET) for the planning of radiotherapy in lung cancer: high impact in patients with atelectasis. Int J Radiat Oncol Biol Phys. 1999;44(3):593–7.
6. Antoch G, Saoudi N, Kuehl H, et al. Accuracy of whole-body dual-modality fluorine-18-2-fluoro-2-deoxy-D-glucose positron emission tomography and computed tomography (FDG-PET/CT) for tumor staging in solid tumors: comparison with CT and PET. J Clin Oncol. 2004;22(21):4357–68.
7. Bentzen SM, Gregoire V. Molecular imaging-based dose painting: a novel paradigm for radiation therapy prescription. Semin Radiat Oncol. 2011;21(2):101–10.
8. McConathy J, Goodman MM. Non-natural amino acids for tumor imaging using positron emission tomography and single photon emission computed tomography. Cancer Metastasis Rev. 2008;27(4):555–73.
9. Pauwels EK, Ribeiro MJ, Stoot JH, McCready VR, Bourguignon M, Maziere B. FDG accumulation and tumor biology. Nucl Med Biol. 1998;25(4):317–22.
10. Reshef A, Shirvan A, Akselrod-Ballin A, Wall A, Ziv I. Small-molecule biomarkers for clinical PET imaging of apoptosis. J Nucl Med. 2010;51(6):837–40.
11. Oborski MJ, Laymon CM, Lieberman FS, Drappatz J, Hamilton RL, Mountz JM. First use of (18)F-labeled ML-10 PET to assess apoptosis change in a newly diagnosed glioblastoma multiforme patient before and early after therapy. Brain Behav. 2014;4(2):312–5.
12. Tehrani OS, Shields AF. PET imaging of proliferation with pyrimidines. J Nucl Med. 2013;54(6):903–12.
13. Haubner R. PET radiopharmaceuticals in radiation treatment planning—synthesis and biological characteristics. Radiother Oncol. 2010;96(3):280–7.
14. Grassi I, Nanni C, Allegri V, et al. The clinical use of PET with (11)C-acetate. Am J Nucl Med Mol Imaging. 2012;2(1):33–47.
15. Virgolini I, Ambrosini V, Bomanji JB, et al. Procedure guidelines for PET/CT tumour imaging with 68Ga-DOTA-conjugated peptides: 68Ga-DOTA-TOC, 68Ga-DOTA-NOC, 68Ga-DOTA-TATE. Eur J Nucl Med Mol Imaging. 2010;37(10):2004–10.
16. Giraud P, Elles S, Helfre S, et al. Conformal radiotherapy for lung cancer: different delineation of the gross tumor volume (GTV) by radiologists and radiation oncologists. Radiother Oncol. 2002;62(1):27–36.
17. Foster B, Bagci U, Mansoor A, Xu Z, Mollura DJ. A review on segmentation of positron emission tomography images. Comput Biol Med. 2014;50:76–96.
18. Cheebsumon P, Boellaard R, de Ruysscher D, et al. Assessment of tumour size in PET/CT lung cancer studies: PET- and CT-based methods compared to pathology. Eur J Nucl Med Mol Imaging. 2012;2(1):56.
19. Frings V, Van Velden FH, Velasquez LM, et al. Repeatability of metabolically active tumor volume measurements with FDG PET/CT in advanced gastrointestinal malignancies: a multicenter study. Radiology. 2014;273(2):539–48.
20. Thorwarth D, Leibfarth S, Monnich D. Potential role of PET/MRI in radiotherapy planning. Clin Transl Imaging. 2013;1:45–51.

Part II

PET/CT in Radiotherapy Planning - Technical and Practical Aspects

Instrumentation

2

Alex Dunlop

Content

References.. 16

Due to recent improvements in radiotherapy treatment planning and delivery, we are now able to generate and deliver highly conformal and homogenous dose distributions to designated targets whilst sparing organs at risks (OARs) [1]. However, the ability to accurately delineate the clinical target volume (CTV) remains one of the major challenges of radiotherapy treatment [2]. Currently, it is standard practice to delineate the CTV on a CT data-set, whilst other imaging modalities may be used to aid the localisation of the target. Functional PET images enable the metabolic activity and extent of the target to be assessed [3].

A single-scan PET/CT approach (Fig. 2.1a) enables the radiotherapy plan to be generated on the CT data-set acquired alongside the PET [4]. This can reduce both the hospital visits for the patient and the image registration uncertainty between the PET image and the radiotherapy planning CT [4]. Indeed, a maximum three-dimensional displacement error between the CT and PET of 0.5 mm has been reported for single-gantry PET/CT systems [5].

To ensure that tumour volumes can be targeted and OARs spared with acceptable accuracy, the position of the patient must remain consistent and reproducible on a daily basis throughout the entire treatment pathway. In order to be able to plan directly from PET/CT data, it is therefore necessary to adapt the PET/CT suite so that patients can be imaged in the treatment position.

Soft-mattress couches commonly used for PET scans (Fig. 2.1b) are not used for radiotherapy treatment; instead flat-top rigid couches are employed to improve

---

A. Dunlop
Department of Physics, The Royal Marsden NHS Foundation Trust, London, UK
e-mail: Alex.dunlop@rmh.nhs.uk

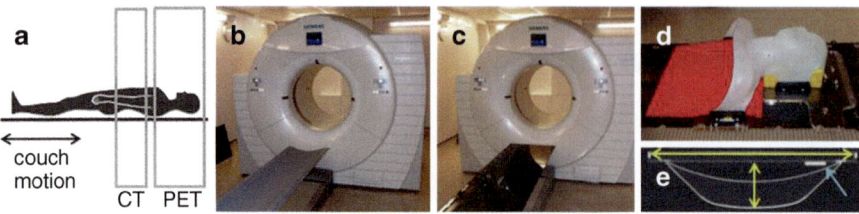

Fig. 2.1 *From left* (**a**) schematic of a single-gantry PET/CT system; (**b**) a Siemens Biograph PET/CT system with diagnostic imaging soft-mattress couch; (**c**) the same PET/CT suite but with a flat radiotherapy couch installed; (**d**) thermoplastic shell attached to the PET/CT flat-top couch using the same immobilisation devices used for radiotherapy treatment—see Chap. 3 for detailed information regarding patient set-up and immobilisation; and (**e**) an axial CT slice of the couch as used for QA—the *yellow arrows* indicate separations that could be measured at regular intervals to check the absolute distance of the CT scanner. Markers of known separation should also be present in the longitudinal direction. The *turquoise arrow* points to a feature of the couch that enables confirmation of left/right sides in the CT image

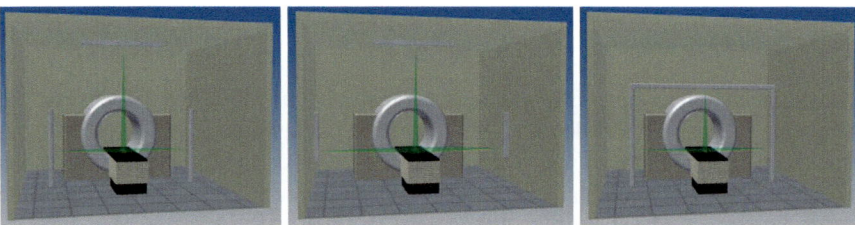

Fig. 2.2 Various commercially available radiotherapy laser systems that could be used within a PET/CT suite, *from left*; free-standing columns for lateral lasers; wall-mounted lateral and sagittal lasers; and a bridge laser arrangement

patient position reproducibility. Therefore, radiotherapy-ready PET/CT systems must be able to easily mount flat-top radiotherapy couches (Fig. 2.1c). The couch top must be consistent with those used for treatment and, in particular, must be compatible with additional immobilisation devices that will be used during treatment. Such devices vary depending on the site of treatment. For example, a patient-specific thermoplastic shell may be used for a head and neck cancer patient (Fig. 2.1d). The flat-top couch should ideally contain markers at known distances from each other (Fig. 2.1e) to allow absolute distance quality assurance (QA) checks to be made at regular intervals in both the longitudinal and lateral directions.

To be used for radiotherapy planning, the PET/CT suite must also incorporate a dedicated radiotherapy laser system. The intersection of the lateral and sagittal lasers determines localisation coordinates within the immobilised patient from which the isocentre for treatment can be defined. The laser system should be consistent with that used on the treatment unit. However, equipment within the PET/CT suite may determine the laser system options that are available (Fig. 2.2). Routine QA must be carried out on the laser system in order to maintain consistency with the lasers in the treatment room. A further consideration is the colour of the laser light. Usually red or green lasers are used; both have the same accuracy and are similar in

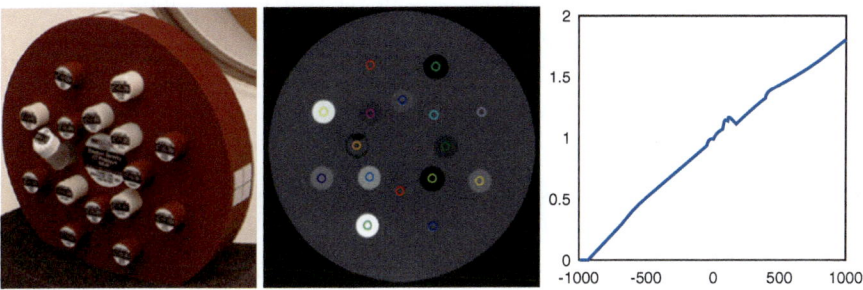

Fig. 2.3 (*Left*) Electron density CT phantom RMI 467 (Gammex, Middleton, WI) in bore of PET/CT scanner. The phantom consists of a solid-water disc the size of an average pelvis with 16 holes in which inserts of differing densities can be placed; (*Middle*) axial CT slice of the RMI phantom viewed within the Pinnacle^3 (Philips, Fitchburg, WI) radiotherapy treatment planning system (TPS). The different inserts have been contoured (various colours) in order to determine the average Hounsfield units (HUs) for each material within the phantom; (*Right*) the resulting scanner-specific plot of physical density (g/cm^3 on the y-axis) as a function of CT number (HU - 1000 on the x-axis)

cost [6]. However, green lasers are known to be more visible on darker skins [6], whereas red lasers are better when aligning patients immobilised within thermoplastic shells. Therefore, careful consideration is needed in the choice of laser colour, particularly in the context of PET/CT where efficiency of patient set-up is important to ensure staff doses are kept as low as reasonably practicable (ALARP).

In order to calculate dose, radiotherapy treatment planning systems (TPSs) require conversion of all voxels in the CT scan from CT numbers or Hounsfield units (HUs) to physical density (g/cm^3). To achieve this, a scanner-specific HU-density look-up table (LUT) is generated and stored within the TPS. The calibration of CT numbers to material density can be realised by performing a CT acquisition on the scanner to be calibrated, using the same scanning parameters to be used for patient scans, of a phantom with various inserts of differing, and known, physical densities. An example of a commercially available phantom capable of defining the calibration is shown in Fig. 2.3. Regular QA should be performed on the CT images to ensure constancy of CT numbers within the image. This can practically be achieved by regularly scanning a phantom of known density and interrogating the resulting image to ensure the CT numbers are as expected.

> **Key Points**
>
> - The ability to accurately delineate the clinical target volume (CTV) remains one of the major challenges of radiotherapy treatment, the use of PET images can aid this process.
> - A single-scan PET/CT approach for radiotherapy treatment planning enables the radiotherapy plan to be generated on the CT data-set acquired alongside the PET, thereby reducing the image registration uncertainty between the two image sets.

- If a single-scan PET/CT acquisition is to be used directly for radiotherapy treatment planning it is vital that the necessary instrumentation is in place to ensure that the patient can be scanned in the treatment position and that localisation can be performed in the same way as on the treatment unit.
- It is vital that a flat-top couch can be easily mounted and that the couch is able to accommodate patient immobilisation systems.
- Radiotherapy-quality laser systems should be installed and tested regularly. Additionally, measurements need to be taken to generate a look-up-table between CT numbers and physical density.

References

1. Otto K. Volumetric modulated arc therapy: IMRT in a single gantry arc. Med Phys. 2008;35(1):310–7.
2. Njeh C. Tumor delineation: the weakest link in the search for accuracy in radiotherapy. J Med Phys. 2008;33(4):136–40.
3. Chiti A, et al. Clinical use of PET/CT data for radiotherapy planning: what are we looking for? Radiother Oncol. 2010;96:277–9.
4. Sattler B, Lee J, Lonsdale M, Coche E. PET/CT (and CT) instrumentation, image reconstruction and data transfer for radiotherapy planning. Radiother Oncol. 2010;96:288–97.
5. Geworski L, et al. Verification of co-registration accuracy of PET/CT [Uberprufung der Co-Registrierung der PET/CT-Daten im Rahmen der Konstanzprufung]. Nuklearmedizin. 2008;47:A83–4.
6. Cherry P, Duxbury A. Practical radiotherapy: physics and equipment. Oxford: Wiley-Blackwell; 2009. p. 202.

Patient Preparation

3

Clare Ockwell and Shirley Summers

Contents

3.1 Patient Positioning.. 20
3.2 Other Considerations... 21
References... 22

When performing a therapy PET/CT scan, efficient and effective communication between the various teams and the patient is essential. Each modality has its own specific patient preparation, and these need to be combined to ensure that both the PET scan and the CT scan are of the best diagnostic quality (or optimal image quality) for radiotherapy planning. Communication and planning is essential prior to the injection of the radioactive tracer used in PET/CT to minimise the patient's anxiety and radiation dose to all staff members (Table 3.1).

The patient preparation for PET/CT scans will depend on the radiotracer being used for the scan. The most commonly used tracer at present is the glucose analogue FDG ($[^{18}F]$ fluorodeoxyglucose). FDG accumulation in tissue is proportional to the amount of glucose utilisation. Increase consumption of glucose is a characteristic of most cancers and is in part related to our expression of the GLUT-1 glucose transporters and hexokinase activity. However, over the last decade, more and more PET radiopharmaceuticals are entering clinics.

Below is a table of different types of tracers used and their uptake mechanism and organs of highest physiological uptake [3] and what preparations are required for each scan (Table 3.2).

C. Ockwell
Department of Radiotherapy, The Royal Marsden NHS Foundation Trust, London, UK

S. Summers (✉)
Nuclear Medicine and PET/CT Department, The Royal Marsden NHS Foundation Trust, London, UK
e-mail: Shirley.summers@rmh.nhs.uk

© Springer International Publishing Switzerland 2017
S. Chua (ed.), *PET/CT in Radiotherapy Planning*, Clinicians' Guides to Radionuclide Hybrid Imaging - PET/CT, DOI 10.1007/978-3-319-54744-2_3

Table 3.1 Patient preparation table combined for all studies

	PET/CT*	Radiotherapy planning CT with contrast
Fasting preparation	√	√
Blood glucose level below 7 mmol/l (140 mg/dl) [1]	√	
Patient changed into hospital gown. Remove all jewellery/metallic objects	√	√
Able to lie still on back for between 20 and 30 min in radiotherapy treatment position	√	√
Kidney function eGFR >60 ml/min/1.73m² or serum creatinine and urea within normal range [2]		√
Not allergic to contrast allergy		√
Not be claustrophobic	√	√

*Please refer to Table 3.2. for specific tracer preparations.

Table 3.2 Current Tracers used in PET/CT scanning with their uptake mechanism and organs of highest physiological uptake and preparations required for scanning

Molecular uptake mechanism	Tracer	Isotope	Organs of highest physiological uptake	Patient fasting preparation
Amino acid transport and protein synthesis	Methionine	F-18	Liver, salivary glands, lachrymal glands, bone marrow, pancreas, bowels, renal cortical, urinary bladder	Fasting for 4–6 h prior to administration [4]. Patient must be well hydrated
	Flouroethyltyrosine	F-18	Pancreas, kidneys, liver, heart, brain, colon, muscle	Patients are not required to fast
	FDOPA	F-18	Pancreas, liver, duodenum, kidneys, gallbladder, biliary duct	Patients are not required to fast
Glucose metabolism	FDG	F-18	Brain, myocardium, breast, liver, spleen, stomach, intestine, kidney, urinary bladder, skeletal muscle, lymphatic tissue, bone marrow, salivary glands, thymus, uterus, ovaries, testicle, brown fat	Fasting preparation of 6 h. Blood glucose level is measured before FDG injection. The ideal glucose level is generally accepted to be lower than 140 mg/dl [1]
				Rest and quiet and warm during uptake period
				Patient must be well hydrated

Table 3.2 (continued)

Molecular uptake mechanism	Tracer	Isotope	Organs of highest physiological uptake	Patient fasting preparation
Proliferation	FLT	F-18	Bone marrow, intestine, kidneys, urinary bladder, liver	Fasting for 4–6 h prior to administration
Hypoxia	FMISO	F-18	Kidney, urinary excretion	Patients are not required to fast
	FAZA	F-18	Kidneys, gall bladder, liver, colon	Patients are not required to fast
	Cu-ATSM	Cu-64	Liver, kidneys, spleen, gall bladder	Patients are not required to fast
Lipid metabolism	Choline	C-11	Liver, pancreas, spleen, salivary glands, lachrymal glands, renal excretion, bone marrow, intestine	Fasting for 4–6 h prior to administration
	Fluoroethylcholine	F-18	Liver, kidneys, salivary glands, urinary bladder, bone marrow, spleen	Fasting for 4–6 h prior to administration
	Acetate	C-11	Gastrointestinal tract, prostate, bone marrow, kidneys, liver, spleen, pancreas	Patients are not required to fast
Angiogenesis/ integrin binding	Galacto-RGD	F-18	Bladder, kidneys, spleen, liver	Patients are not required to fast but should not have impaired renal function (serum creatinine level > 1.2 mg/dl) [5]
	AH111585	F-18	Bladder, liver, intestine, kidneys	
SSTR binding	DOTATOC	Ga-68	Pituitary and adrenal glands, pancreas, spleen, urinary bladder, liver, thyroid	Fasting is not necessary. It has been recommended that octreotide therapy be discontinued (1 day) for short-lived molecules and 3–4 weeks for long-acting analogues [6]
	DOTATATE	Ga-68	Spleen, urinary bladder, liver	

Fasting Preparations for Patients with Diabetes Mellitus [1]:

Type II diabetes mellitus (controlled by oral medication):

The PET scan should be performed in the late morning, and patients must comply with the fasting instructions as indicated above. Patients continue to take oral medication to control their blood sugar.

Type I diabetes mellitus and insulin-dependant type II diabetes mellitus:

Ideally an attempt should be made to achieve normal glycaemic values prior to the PET study. The PET study should be scheduled for the late morning. The patient should eat a normal breakfast (4 h prior to administration of PET tracer) and inject the normal amount of insulin. Thereafter the patient should not eat any more food or fluid apart from tap water.

3.1 Patient Positioning

Ideally patient position for radiotherapy planning should be established and set up before the administration of the radioactive tracer. Patients should be positioned on a flat carbon fibre couch top in the radiotherapy planning position where possible. This requires the use of immobilisation devices and externally mounted lasers. These devices depend on the anatomical region to be treated according to local radiotherapy protocols (see Table 3.3).

These devices should be positioned and attached to the flat couch top using a location bar at the appropriate index position for scanning purposes. All patient positions need to be carefully documented. Following the positioning session, the patient should be injected with the tracer in an alternative room for the appropriate time. The patient should be repositioned with the radiotherapy team and nuclear medicine team working closely together using the external lasers where present to align the tattoos/reference points to reproduce the patient position accurately; this requires manipulation of the patient position on the couch to align the tattoos/reference points.

Table 3.3 Patient positioning

Anatomical site	Typical radiotherapy position and immobilisation
Brain	Supine, thermoplastic mask (head only), head and neck board, head rest and additional supportive pads
Head and neck	Supine, thermoplastic mask (head and shoulders), head and neck board, head rest and additional supportive knee pad
Thorax and abdomen	Supine, arms up, lung board, knee pad
Breast	Supine, both arms or one arm up, inclined board up to 15° with arm supports
Pelvis	Supine or prone, knee and lower leg and foot immobilisation device, supportive pad under head

PET/CT scanning protocols should include the target volume plus a margin of surrounding anatomy. Once PET/CT has been acquired, it can be followed by a contrast enhanced CT for planning purposes; scanning levels should include the target volume and organs at risk relative to the volume to be treated in their entirety according to local radiotherapy protocols. Tattoos and reference marks should be highlighted with the use of radiopaque CT markers.

3.2   Other Considerations

It may be advisable to reserve specific camera time for these planning PET/CT scans. This would allow members of the radiotherapy team to attend the department to assist set up patients for the PET/CT scans. Radiotherapy staff needs to be issued with sounding dosimeters and have sufficient training regarding radiation protection in respect to PET/CT patients. The reservation of PET/CT cameras and inclusion of radiotherapy staff will have recourse implications which need to be carefully considered before undertaking this service.

Key Points

- When performing a therapy PET/CT scan, efficient and effective communication between the various teams and the patient is essential.
- The patient preparation for PET/CT scans will depend on the radiotracer being used for the scan.
- The most commonly used tracer at present is the glucose analogue 18F-FDG.
- Ideally patient position for radiotherapy planning should be established and set up before the administration of the radioactive tracer.
- All patient positions need to be carefully documented.
- PET/CT scanning protocols should include the target volume plus a margin of surrounding anatomy.
- PET/CT scanning can be followed by a contrast enhanced CT for planning purposes; scanning levels should include the target volume and organs at risk relative to the volume to be treated in their entirety according to local radiotherapy protocols.
- Tattoos and reference marks should be highlighted with the use of radiopaque CT markers.
- Reserve specific camera time for these planning PET/CT scans.

References

1. Ronald B, O'Doherty MJ, Weber WA, Mottaghy FM, Lonsdale MN, Stroobants SG, Oyen WJG, Kotzerke J, Hoekstra OS, Pruim J, Marsden PK, Tatsch K, Hoekstra CJ, Visser EP, Arends B, Verzijlbergen FJ, Zijlstra JM, Comans EFI, Lammertsma AA, Paans AM, Willemsen AT, Beyer T, Bockisch A, Schaefer-Prokop C, Delbeke D, Baum RP, Chiti A, Krause BJ. FDG PET and PET/CT: EANM procedure guidelines for tumour PET imaging: version 1.0. Eur J Nucl Med Mol Imaging. 2010;37(1):181–200.
2. The Royal College of Radiologists. Standards for intravascular contrast agent administration to adult patients. 2nd ed. London: Royal College of Radiologists; 2010.
3. Haubner R. PET radiopharmaceuticals in radiation treatment planning—synthesis and biological characteristics. Radiother Oncol. 2010;96:280–7.
4. Nuñez R, Macapinlac HA, Yeung HW, Akhurst T, Cai S, Osman I, Gonen M, Riedel E, Scher HI, Larson SM. Combined 18F-FDG and 11C-Methionine PET scans in patients with newly progressive metastatic prostate cancer. J Nucl Med. 2002;43(1):46–55.
5. Schnell O, Krebs B, Carlsen J, Miederer I, Goetz C, Goldbrunner RH, Wester H-J, Haubner R, Pöpperl G, Holtmannspötter M, Kretzschmar HA, Kessler H, Tonn J-C, Schwaiger M, Beer AJ. Imaging of integrin $\alpha v \beta 3$ expression in patients with malignant glioma by [18F] Galacto-RGD positron emission tomography. Neuro Oncol. 2009;11(6):861–70.
6. Taïeb D, Timmers HJ, Hindié E, Guillet BA, Neumann HP, Walz MK, Opocher G, de Herder WW, Boedeker CC, de Krijger RR, Chiti A, Al-Nahhas A, Pacak K, Rubello D. EANM 2012 guidelines for radionuclide imaging of phaeochromocytoma and paraganglioma. Eur J Nucl Med Mol Imaging. 2012;39:1977–95.

Data Acquisition, Reconstruction and Transfer

4

David Towey and Laurence Hill

Contents

4.1	PET Acquisition and Reconstruction: Standard Options in PET Scanning...	23
4.2	Deviation for RT Planning PET...	24
4.3	CT Acquisition: Standard Options in Diagnostic Scanning	24
4.4	Deviation for RT Planning CT..	24
4.5	Respiratory Gating..	25
4.6	DICOM, DICOM-RT and Other Options	25
References...		27

4.1 PET Acquisition and Reconstruction: Standard Options in PET Scanning

The majority of clinical PET/CT scanning is performed using 2-deoxy-2-(^{18}F)fluoro-D-glucose (FDG) in whole or 'half' body scans. These take the form of full-image sweeps from below the orbits to midway down the thigh. Most scanners acquire the data as a series of overlapping static views (or bed positions) which are then combined to produce a single continuous volume of data. The data recorded from the PET scanner is in the form of sinogram data. This needs to be reconstructed to produce the transverse slices which make up the complete volume. Various methodologies for reconstruction exist and are an active area of research [1]. Such a broad range of methodologies necessarily leads to a wide variation of image characteristics (including noise, resolution and quantitative accuracy metrics). Strategies for standardisation have been suggested [2–4] which all modern scanners can easily achieve but may fall short of the imaging performance that can be achieved with these systems.

D. Towey (✉) • L. Hill
Radiological Sciences Unit, Imperial College Healthcare NHS Trust, London, UK
e-mail: david.towey@ngh.nhs.uk

Guidelines for clinical ^{18}F-FDG vary in recommendations for administered activity—SNM guidelines quote a range of 370–740 MBq [5] but are not prescriptive, whereas the EANM guidelines [3] suggest a weight-based scaling which typically produce activities in the range 200–450 MBq, but this varies with technology used and scan speed. The BNMS guidelines mirror the EANM recommendations, and the ARSAC [6] guidelines set a maximum injected activity of 400 MBq for a standard-sized patient, which they refer to as a diagnostic reference level.

4.2 Deviation for RT Planning PET

Clinical PET scanning is a trade-off between image quality and patient dose, patient comfort and likelihood of patient motion. If immobilisation devices are used (see Chap. 2), it is possible to scan specific areas with increased acquisition times—typically 10 mins—which can lead to better quality PET images. It may be possible to use less smoothing in the reconstruction with the improved count statistics, and the reconstruction settings should be optimised for these images.

4.3 CT Acquisition: Standard Options in Diagnostic Scanning

In PET/CT imaging, the CT dataset is used for attenuation correction of the PET data, anatomical localisation of any lesions seen on the PET and depending on the quality of the CT images for direct clinical evaluation. In most diagnostic PET/CT scanning, the CT doses are optimised as relatively low-dose procedures with associated lower diagnostic utility. These AC-CT acquisitions typically involve a single continuous exposure with uniform slicing and reconstruction settings throughout. Tube current modulation can be employed to improve the dose/image quality optimisation. These scans result in effective doses of around 5–10 mSv for a half body scan which is approximately 1/3 of the dose from the equivalent clinical CT examination.

4.4 Deviation for RT Planning CT

There are a number of options for the CT component as it can be used for three distinct purposes:

- The CT data is scaled to produce the electron density map on which the dose distributions are calculated.
- Treatment volumes of interest (both targets and organs of risk) can be defined using high-quality CT data with or without contrast
- The AC-CT can be used to co-register the PET data with other CT datasets.

For the first two uses, the CT data has to be of sufficient quality to allow good-quality planning to occur. Suitable image quality is certainly achievable using current clinical PET/CT scanners, but limitations in workflows and acquisition details will generally require them to be acquired as secondary acquisitions taken after the routine whole/half body acquisition for the PET/CT.

Thus the option for 'one-stop' acquisition of the PET/CT and planning data is unlikely to give any significant dose saving as both low-dose full body scanning and high-quality localised CT will both be required. Depending of patient pathways and availability of scanning slots, there may still be an advantage to performing all on a single day.

The handling of CT contrast by the RT planning system varies by centre and can include dual acquisition or image correction. There is also evidence to show that the error in the resulting therapy plan may not be clinically significant [7].

For the AC-CT data to be co-registered with the radiotherapy CT dataset, it is best if the PET study is performed on a flat couch top and, for head and neck studies, with the patient position fixed in the head cast system. This requires that the PET/CT be equipped with the same fixation devices as used in radiotherapy and the laser alignment system to allow accurate patient positioning. See Chap. 2.

4.5 Respiratory Gating

The use of respiratory gating in both PET and radiotherapy application has been an area of research for many years and is now starting to be implemented clinically. If treatments are to be given in a respiratory gated form, then planning data must also be gated. However, the approach in PET is to normalise to the end expiration which would have to be adjusted to end inspiration to match RT techniques.

4.6 DICOM, DICOM-RT and Other Options

The Digital Imaging and Communications in Medicine (DICOM) standard is an internationally used system for distributing and viewing medical image data. It was introduced to allow cross-vendor distraction of image data and allowed the near universal introduction of PACS systems. Within the DICOM standard, there are many modality-specific attributes (or TAGs) which can be used to include important information about the image dataset to allow proper processing, analysis and interpretation. These include basic image details such as pixel and matrix sizes, pixel scaling details and in the case of PET data the scaling factors needed to convert the pixel data into SUV figures.

Key Points

- Various methodologies for reconstruction exist and are an active area of research.
- Strategies for standardisation have been suggested, which all modern scanners can easily achieve.
- Guidelines for clinical ^{18}F-FDG vary in recommendations for administered activity.
- Clinical PET scanning is a trade-off between image quality and patient dose, patient comfort and likelihood of patient motion.
- In PET/CT imaging, the CT dataset is used for attenuation correction of the PET data, anatomical localisation of any lesions seen on the PET and depending on the quality of the CT images for direct clinical evaluation.
- In most diagnostic PET/CT scanning, the CT doses are optimised as relatively low-dose procedures with associated lower diagnostic utility.
- There are a number of options for the CT component as it can be used for three distinct purposes.
  - The CT data is scaled to produce the electron density map on which the dose distributions are calculated.
  - Treatment volumes of interest (both targets and organs of risk) can be defined using high-quality CT data with or without contrast.
  - The AC-CT can be used to co-register the PET data with other CT datasets.
- The handling of CT contrast by the RT planning system varies by centre and can include dual acquisition or image correction.
- For the AC-CT data to be co-registered with the radiotherapy CT dataset, it is best if the PET study is performed on a flat couch top and, for head and neck studies, with the patient position fixed in the head cast system.
- The use of respiratory gating in both PET and radiotherapy application has been an area of research for many years and is now starting to be implemented clinically. If treatments are to be given in a respiratory-gated form, then planning data must also be gated.

An addition set attributes allow the DICOM standard to be utilised in the various stages of radiotherapy treatments. Collectively known as 'DICOM-RT', these include sections on image, dose, structures sets, plan information and treatment records. The structure-set object includes information about treatment target volumes and organs of interest. Some PACS systems are not configured to process these added fields which must be considered if volumes are being defined on the PET system. Direct PET-RT transfer is generally less problematic in this respect assuming such a network connection can be made.

References

1. Hutton BF. Recent advances in iterative reconstruction for clinical SPECT/PET and CT. Acta Oncol. 2011;50:851–8.
2. British Nuclear Medicine Society (BNMS) Combined procedure guidelines of SNM, EANM and BNMS for SPECT/CT and PETCT imaging. 2013. www.bnms.org.uk/procedures-guidelines/bnms-clinical-guidelines/procedure-guidelines-for-spectct-and-petct-imaging.html. Accessed 20 Oct 2014.
3. Boellaard R, O'Doherty MJ, Weber WA, Mottaghy FM, Lonsdale MN, Stroobants SG, Oyen WJ, Kotzerke J, Hoekstra OS, Pruim J, Marsden PK, Tatsch K, Hoekstra CJ, Visser EP, Arends B, Verzijlbergen FJ, Zijlstra JM, Comans EF, Lammertsma AA, Paans AM, Willemsen AT, Beyer T, Bockisch A, Schaefer-Prokop C, Delbeke D, Baum RP, Chiti A, Krause BJ. FDG PET and PET/CT: EANM procedure guidelines for tumour PET imaging: version 1.0. Eur J Nucl Med Mol Imaging. 2010;37(1):181–200. doi:10.1007/s00259-009-1297-4.
4. Institute of Physics and Engineering in Medicine (IPEM) report 108. Quality assurance of PET and PET/CT systems. 2013.
5. Boellaard R. Standards for PET image acquisition and quantitative data analysis. J Nucl Med. 2009;50:11S–20S.
6. ARSAC. Notes for guidance on the clinical administration of radiopharmaceuticals and use of sealed radioactive sources. 2014. www.arsac.org.uk. Accessed 20 Oct 2014.
7. Choi Y, Kim J, Lee H, et al. Influence of intravenous contrast agent on dose calculations of intensity modulated radiation therapy plans for head and neck cancer. Radiother Oncol. 2006;81:158–62.

Sources of Artefacts: Consequences and Solutions

5

Alison Tree and Maria Hawkins

Content

References... 32

While PET shows much promise in improving target delineation in radiotherapy planning, there are some pitfalls which must be acknowledged before adopting wholescale implementation.

State-of-the-art PET/CT scanners are recommended for radiotherapy planning. A bore size of 70 cm (accommodates RT immobilization devices and large patients) is preferred. An integrated CT scanner with flat couch and contrast facilities would permit the use of CT component of the PET for RT planning.

There are several artefacts (Table 5.1) encountered in PET/CT imaging which can mimic FDG-avid malignant lesions, and therefore recognition of these artefacts is clinically relevant and has implications when SUV is used to derive region of interest used for planning.

CT imaging with intravenous contrast, as a component of the exam, can cause challenges as it mimics intense FDG uptake [1, 2]. A simple solution to resolving the uncertainty is to inspect the non-attenuated correction PET images or to perform a low-dose non-contrast CT prior to contrast administration.

Metallic objects such as dental fillings [3], orthopedic devices, and fiducial markers can demonstrate falsely elevated tracer uptake. The high CT number of metal can result in overestimation of the SUV.

A. Tree (✉)
Royal Marsden NHS Foundation Trust and the Institute of Cancer Research, London, SW3 6JJ, UK
e-mail: Alison.tree@rmh.nhs.uk

M. Hawkins
CRUK MRC Oxford Institute for Radiation Oncology, Gray Laboratories, University of Oxford, Oxford, OX3 7DQ, UK

© Springer International Publishing Switzerland 2017
S. Chua (ed.), *PET/CT in Radiotherapy Planning*, Clinicians' Guides to Radionuclide Hybrid Imaging - PET/CT, DOI 10.1007/978-3-319-54744-2_5

Table 5.1 Examples of artefact in PET/CT

PET-based errors	Errors from CT-based attenuation
Calibration problems	CT artefacts
Detector failures	Non-biological objects in patients[a]
Resolution and partial volume effects[a]	Respiratory mismatch between PET and CT images[a]
Patient motion[a]	Patient motion[a]
Non-malignant FDG avidity[a]	

[a]Artifacts that can cause specific problems for RT planning

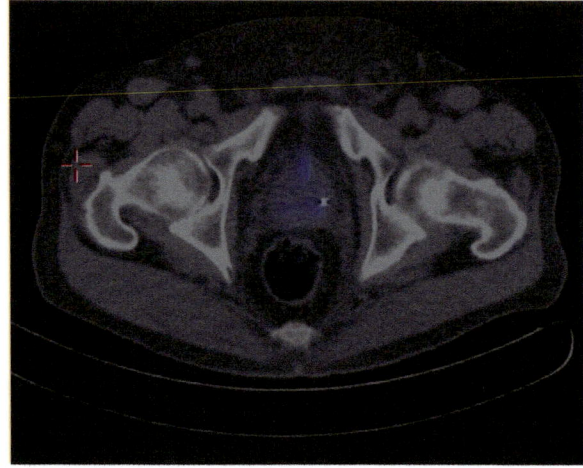

Fig. 5.1 Nonmalignant choline PET uptake in the prostate around fiducial markers

In addition, there are many nonmalignant processes which can mimic tumor on PET such as inflammation around a stent [4], benign inflammation of an organ such as prostatitis [5] (see Fig. 5.1), and postsurgical changes.

The field of view of a standard CT is 50 cm, whereas PET imagers can detect a field around 70 cm wide. This leads to truncation, a lack of ability to correct the lateral aspects of the PET for CT attenuation. This can artefactually reduce SUV.

In areas where there is a large change in attenuation over a small distance, potentially artefactual uptake can be seen with small errors in fusion. This can be reduced by scanning in a radiotherapy immobilization device and/or laser alignment. Reports on 3D displacements between CT and PET indicate a displacement error of 0.5 mm [6].

Respiratory motion remains the main challenge for RT planning of lung [7] and upper GI tract [8] malignancies. The misalignment between scans is most noticeable at the left lung and in the bases [6, 9, 10] and upper abdomen (hepatic area) [11].

In addition to image registration mismatch, respiratory motion can lead to a decrease of FDG concentration in (lung) tumors [12]. Erdi et al. describes lesion displacements of 6.4–24.7 mm when 4DCT was registered with PET which correlates with a decrease in tumor SUV of 6–24% between the extremes of the respiratory cycle [13].

Different strategies to reduce respiratory motion artifacts have been proposed including breathing coaching; exhale breathhold has been suggested to be the best option as this is reproducible and permits a reduction of breathing artifacts up to 28% when compared with free-breathing scans [14]. Deep inspiratory breathhold was proposed by Nehmeh et al. [15]. These techniques are all dependent on patient compliance.

4D PET/CT is discussed in Chap. 7.

Knowledge of potential sources of artefacts and awareness of the potential advantages and disadvantages of intervention has the potential to produce better quality PET/CT images that may improve the target volume delineation for PET guided RT.

Key Points

- State-of-the-art PET/CT scanners are recommended for radiotherapy planning.
- A bore size of 70 cm (accommodates RT immobilization devices and large patients) is preferred.
- An integrated CT scanner with flat couch and contrast facilities would permit the use of CT component of the PET for RT planning.
- There are several artefacts encountered in PET/CT imaging which can mimic FDG-avid malignant lesions, and therefore recognition of these artefacts is clinically relevant and has implications when SUV is used to derive region of interest used for planning.
- CT imaging with intravenous contrast, as a component of the exam, can cause challenges as it mimics intense FDG uptake. A simple solution to resolving the uncertainty is to (a) inspect the non-attenuated correction PET images or (b) to perform a low-dose non-contrast CT prior to contrast administration.
- Metallic objects such as dental fillings, orthopedic devices, and fiducial markers can demonstrate falsely elevated tracer uptake (high CT number of metal can result in overestimation of the SUV).
- The field of view of a standard CT is 50 cm, whereas PET imagers can detect a field around 70 cm wide. This leads to truncation, a lack of ability to correct the lateral aspects of the PET for CT attenuation. This can artifactually reduce SUV.
- Respiratory motion remains the main challenge for RT planning of lung and upper GI tract malignancies. The misalignment between scans is most noticeable at the left lung and in the bases and upper abdomen (hepatic area).
- Knowledge of potential sources of artifacts, advantages, and limitations of intervention can lead to better quality PET/CT images that may improve the target volume delineation for PET guided RT.

References

1. Antoch G, Freudenberg LS, Egelhof T, Stattaus J, Jentzen W, Debatin JF, et al. Focal tracer uptake: a potential artifact in contrast-enhanced dual-modality PET/CT scans. J Nucl Med. 2002;43(10):1339–42.
2. Yau YY, Chan WS, Tam YM, Vernon P, Wong S, Coel M, et al. Application of intravenous contrast in PET/CT: does it really introduce significant attenuation correction error? Journal of nuclear medicine: official publication. J Nucl Med. 2005;46(2):283–91.
3. Goerres GW, Hany TF, Kamel E, von Schulthess GK, Buck A. Head and neck imaging with PET and PET/CT: artefacts from dental metallic implants. Eur J Nucl Med Mol Imaging. 2002;29(3):367–70.
4. Wilson JM, Partridge M, Hawkins M. The application of functional imaging techniques to personalise chemoradiotherapy in upper gastrointestinal malignancies. Clin Oncol (R Coll Radiol). 2014;26(9):581–96.
5. Schwarzenbock S, Souvatzoglou M, Krause BJ. Choline PET and PET/CT in primary diagnosis and staging of prostate cancer. Theranostics. 2012;2(3):318–30.
6. Weigert M, Pietrzyk U, Muller S, Palm C, Beyer T. Whole-body PET/CT imaging: combining software- and hardware-based co-registration. Zeitschrift fur medizinische Physik. 2008;18(1):59–66.
7. Goerres GW, Kamel E, Seifert B, Burger C, Buck A, Hany TF, et al. Accuracy of image coregistration of pulmonary lesions in patients with non-small cell lung cancer using an integrated PET/CT system. J Nucl Med. 2002;43(11):1469–75.
8. Nakamoto Y, Tatsumi M, Cohade C, Osman M, Marshall LT, Wahl RL. Accuracy of image fusion of normal upper abdominal organs visualized with PET/CT. Eur J Nucl Med Mol Imaging. 2003;30(4):597–602.
9. Cohade C, Osman M, Marshall LN, Wahl RN. PET/CT: accuracy of PET and CT spatial registration of lung lesions. Eur J Nucl Med Mol Imaging. 2003;30(5):721–6.
10. Goerres GW, Kamel E, Heidelberg TN, Schwitter MR, Burger C, von Schulthess GK. PET/CT image co-registration in the thorax: influence of respiration. Eur J Nucl Med Mol Imaging. 2002;29(3):351–60.
11. Osman MM, Cohade C, Nakamoto Y, Marshall LT, Leal JP, Wahl RL. Clinically significant inaccurate localization of lesions with PET/CT: frequency in 300 patients. J Nucl Med. 2003;44(2):240–3.
12. Goerres GW, Burger C, Kamel E, Seifert B, Kaim AH, Buck A, et al. Respiration-induced attenuation artifact at PET/CT: technical considerations. Radiology. 2003;226(3):906–10.
13. Erdi YE, Nehmeh SA, Pan T, Pevsner A, Rosenzweig KE, Mageras G, et al. The CT motion quantitation of lung lesions and its impact on PET-measured SUVs. J Nucl Med. 2004;45(8):1287–92.
14. de Juan R, Seifert B, Berthold T, von Schulthess GK, Goerres GW. Clinical evaluation of a breathing protocol for PET/CT. Eur Radiol. 2004;14(6):1118–23.
15. Nehmeh SA, Erdi YE, Meirelles GS, Squire O, Larson SM, Humm JL, et al. Deep-inspiration breath-hold PET/CT of the thorax. J Nucl Med. 2007;48(1):22–6.

Advantages and Limitations

6

Shaista Hafeez and Robert Huddart

Contents

6.1	Introduction	33
6.2	Advantages	33
6.2.1	Accuracy in Disease Delineation	33
6.2.2	Future Potential for Individualizing Radiotherapy Treatment	34
6.3	Considerations and Limitations	35
References		37

6.1 Introduction

CT alone has conventionally informed radiotherapy planning. It provides anatomical information for delineation and electron density for dose calculation. Integrating PET/CT for radiotherapy planning offers the opportunity to individualize treatment and improve patient outcome. PET/CT's molecular insight of tumour biology could facilitate a move away from 'one-size-fits-all' prescription to more accurate personalized radiotherapy [1].

6.2 Advantages

6.2.1 Accuracy in Disease Delineation

PET/CT can more closely reflect pathological staging and improve interobserver concordance of tumour and involved lymph node delineation [2]. Accuracy in

---

S. Hafeez (✉) • R. Huddart
The Royal Marsden NHS Foundation Trust, Downs Road, Sutton, SM2 5PT Surrey, UK

The Institute of Cancer Research, 123 Old Brompton Road, London, SW7 3RP UK
e-mail: Shaista.Hafeez@icr.c.uk

© Springer International Publishing Switzerland 2017
S. Chua (ed.), *PET/CT in Radiotherapy Planning*, Clinicians' Guides
to Radionuclide Hybrid Imaging - PET/CT, DOI 10.1007/978-3-319-54744-2_6

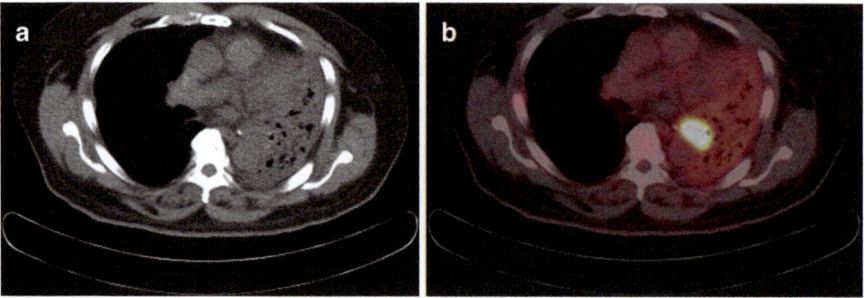

Fig. 6.1 Non-small cell cancer affecting left lung, (**a**) axial slice through radiotherapy planning CT, demonstrating associated collapse and consolidation making tumour boundaries difficult to distinguish, (**b**) FDG-PET/CT axial slice through corresponding area shows FDG avidity of tumour (SUV_{max} 28.8) to guide delineation for radical radiotherapy

contouring is fundamental to ensure dose is delivered to the correct areas. Certainty in tumour delineation often results in smaller treatment volumes with less normal tissue irradiation [3]. As a result PET/CT is commonly used for radical lung radiotherapy planning because of well-known difficulties in distinguishing tumour, necrosis, atelectasis and normal tissue boundaries (Fig. 6.1) [2].

6.2.2 Future Potential for Individualizing Radiotherapy Treatment

PET/CT offers ability to identify biological sub-volumes within the tumour and could be used with intensity-modulated radiotherapy (IMRT) to allow complex dose shaping with non-uniform dose (Fig. 6.2). For example, hypoxic tumour regions demonstrate intrinsic radioresistance, ^{64}Cu-ATSM could be used to define these areas and inform sub-volume for dose escalation [4]. This strategy is known as 'dose painting by contours'; a PET-based volume (biological target volume) is treated to a specified dose level while keeping the mean dose to the remaining target constant. Alternatively quantitative PET information can be used to adapt the radiotherapy prescription. This is known as 'dose painting by numbers', an inhomogeneous dose across the target volume is informed by the PET voxel intensity [5]. Numerous planning studies in various tumour types have shown feasibility of these approaches to inform radiotherapy planning; however randomized clinical trials are needed to demonstrate whether this translates to improving local disease control and toxicity for patients [5].

PET/CT performed during the course of radiotherapy may also facilitate adaptation of the remaining fractions to either increase dose to sub-volumes with apparent

6 Advantages and Limitations

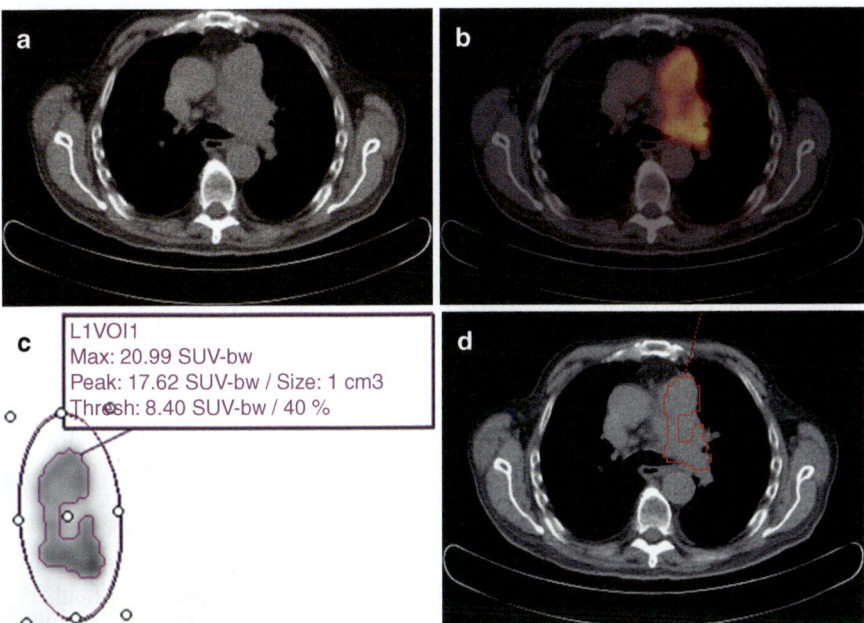

Fig. 6.2 Non-small cell lung cancer of left lung with infiltration of mediastinum, right thoracic inlet and right hilar lymphadenopathy (T4N3), (**a**) axial slice through radiotherapy planning CT, (**b**) FDG-PET/CT axial slice through corresponding area shows heterogeneity of FDG uptake through tumour volume, (**c**) sub-volume for potential dose escalation defined by SUV thresholding, (**d**) region of interest imported into planning system, however, requires further registration optimization for planning purposes

poor response or reduce dose to areas of excellent radiotherapy response to spare normal tissue further.

6.3 Considerations and Limitations

Given that planning CT provides the electron density information from which dose calculations are currently made, PET/CT images require precise registration to the planning CT.

For rigid registration, patient scanning takes place with identical setup to that of radiotherapy planning and treatment, i.e. flat top couch, immobilization devices, light lasers and tattoos as appropriate [6]. Alternatively deformable registration algorithms accommodate for any spatial difference between the volume elements of the different scans [7]. Some setup parameters however may not be possible to reproduce. For example, the PET/CT bore size may prevent the use of some immobilization devices; a full bladder may be indicated for treatment (e.g. prostate) but is avoided for PET/CT to minimize radioactivity bladder accumulation.

Disease sites subject to significant respiratory motion can introduce uncertainty and artefact. As a result the specific uptake value (SUV) may be underestimated or the volume overestimated. For this reason motion mitigation strategies should be considered particularly for thoracic tumours as they are in radiotherapy [7, 8].

Quantitative analysis of the SUV is also subject to a number of other potential errors including extravasation or incomplete injection, longer uptake period and patient's blood glucose in circumstances where ^{18}FDG-PET is used [9].

Contouring with PET/CT can be operator dependent as there are no robust standard for display thresholds. Adjustments to the image windowing settings are often arbitrary and can easily make the tumour appear bigger or smaller introducing a potential systematic error. The alternative is to use automatic or semiautomatic segmentation methods [3]. This also leads to different volumes depending on method used [10].

Dose painting methods are subject to these technical limitations but also from the PET voxel size used, the biological and chemical characteristics of the tracer used and the accuracy of dose calculations with small radiotherapy treatment fields [9]. The technical issues of the accuracy of radiotherapy delivery need to be considered if boosting small volumes particularly if there are significant dose gradients to ensure areas to be boosted receive the intended dose.

The other fundamental issue is that the metabolic state of tumours is likely to be dynamic. So a hypoxic subregion for one fraction may be in a different for the subsequent fractions. This then necessitates more dynamic dose painting approaches.

Conclusion

In practice PET/CT remains an expensive imaging modality with limited wider acceptance in routine clinical planning. The majority of work to date has been dosimetric planning studies, further trials to determine whether this translates into clinical benefit is required. Multicentre trials with PET however face specific issues so require emphasis on standardization and validation of methods to produce meaningful results. In the UK establishing accredited scanning sites operating to rigorous standards is now recognized as the best way to achieve this.

Key Points

- Integrating PET/CT for radiotherapy planning offers the opportunity to individualize treatment and improve patient outcome.
- PET/CT's molecular insight of tumour biology could facilitate a move away from 'one-size-fits-all' prescription to more accurate personalized radiotherapy.

- PET/CT can more closely reflect pathological staging and improve interobserver concordance of tumour and involved lymph node delineation.
- PET/CT is commonly used for radical lung radiotherapy planning because of well-known difficulties in distinguishing tumour, necrosis, atelectasis and normal tissue boundaries.
- PET/CT offers ability to identify biological sub-volumes within the tumour and could be used with intensity-modulated radiotherapy (IMRT) to allow complex dose shaping with non-uniform dose.
- PET/CT performed during the course of radiotherapy may also facilitate adaptation of the remaining fractions to either increase dose to sub-volumes with apparent poor response or reduce dose to areas of excellent radiotherapy response to spare normal tissue further.
- Given that planning CT provides electron density information from which dose calculations are currently made, PET/CT images require precise registration to the planning CT.
- Disease sites subject to significant respiratory motion can introduce uncertainty and artefact (SUV may be underestimated or the volume overestimated).
- Quantitative analysis of the SUV is also subject to a number of other potential errors including extravasation or incomplete injection, longer uptake period and patient's blood glucose in circumstances (where ^{18}FDG-PET is used).
- Contouring with PET/CT can be operator dependent as there are no robust standard for display thresholds.
- Metabolic state of tumours is likely to be dynamic (hypoxic subregion for one fraction may be in a different for the subsequent fractions) and necessitates more dynamic dose painting approaches.

Acknowledgements We acknowledge NHS funding to the NIHR Biomedical Research Centre for Cancer and to Cancer Research UK (CRUK).

Conflict of Interest Notification No conflicts of interest.

References

1. Mankoff DA. A definition of molecular imaging. J Nucl Med. 2007;48(6):18N–21N.
2. De Ruysscher D, Kirsch CM. PET scans in radiotherapy planning of lung cancer. Radiother Oncol. 2010;96(3):335–8.
3. Chiti A, Kirienko M, Gregoire V. Clinical use of PET-CT data for radiotherapy planning: what are we looking for? Radiother Oncol. 2010;96(3):277–9.

4. Hockel M, Schlenger K, Aral B, Mitze M, Schaffer U, Vaupel P. Association between tumor hypoxia and malignant progression in advanced cancer of the uterine cervix. Cancer Res. 1996;56(19):4509–15.
5. Thorwarth D, Geets X, Paiusco M. Physical radiotherapy treatment planning based on functional PET-CT data. Radiother Oncol. 2010;96(3):317–24.
6. Coffey M, Vaandering A. Patient setup for PET-CT acquisition in radiotherapy planning. Radiother Oncol. 2010;96(3):298–301.
7. Scripes PG, Yaparpalvi R. Technical aspects of positron emission tomography/computed tomography in radiotherapy treatment planning. Semin Nucl Med. 2012;42(5):283–8.
8. Bettinardi V, Picchio M, Di Muzio N, Gianolli L, Gilardi MC, Messa C. Detection and compensation of organ/lesion motion using 4D-PET-CT respiratory gated acquisition techniques. Radiother Oncol. 2010;96(3):311–6.
9. Weber WA. Quantitative analysis of PET studies. Radiother Oncol. 2010;96(3):308–10.
10. Nestle U, Schaefer-Schuler A, Kremp S, Groeschel A, Hellwig D, Rube C, Kirsch CM. Target volume definition for 18F-FDG PET-positive lymph nodes in radiotherapy of patients with non-small cell lung cancer. Eur J Nucl Med Mol Imaging. 2007;34(4):453–62.

4D PET/CT Respiratory Gated Acquisition Techniques

Iain Murray

Contents

7.1 Introduction 39
7.2 Breath-Hold Techniques 40
7.3 4D PET/CT 40
References 42

7.1 Introduction

As previously described, the aim of radiotherapy is to deliver a high dose of radiation to a tumour whilst minimising the radiation dose delivered to surrounding tissue. Significant developments in conformal techniques mean that it is increasingly possible to plan and deliver irregular dose distributions that meet these conditions.

However, one of the most important limiting factors affecting radiation delivery is the ability to match the positioning of the radiation beams to the target in question. In order to account for positioning uncertainties, it has become standard practice to add a margin to the defined target [1–3].

The addition of margins clearly reduces the therapeutic index (the relationship between the dose delivered to the tumour and the dose delivered to the surrounding tissue). In situations where there is significant movement of the target tumour, either inter-fractionally over several days or during the seconds/minutes for which the treatment beam is turned on, then the therapeutic index is compromised further.

Respiratory motion will affect all organs within the thorax and abdomen to some degree [4]. Lungs are most affected followed by liver and breast. Therefore a number of strategies have been developed over the last 20 years in order to manage motion and attempt to improve clinical outcomes.

I. Murray
Royal Marsden NHS Trust, The Royal Marsden Hospital, London SW3 6JJ, UK
e-mail: Iain.murray@icr.ac.uk

7.2 Breath-Hold Techniques

One early technique was to focus on breath-hold techniques at both the point of treatment delivery on the linear accelerator and at the point of imaging patients for planning purposes.

Breath-hold CT imaging is relatively easy to accomplish, particularly given the fast acquisition times which modern scanners can achieve. Breath holding can be patient controlled or alternatively undertaken with an active breathing control (ABC) method. ABC devices monitor the patient's respiratory cycle using a valved spirometer and enable a breath-hold at a predetermined point in that cycle.

Typical PET imaging protocols acquire emission data for at least 2 min per bed position. None the less, there have been several investigations into breath-hold PET imaging [5–8]. Imaging is generally limited to a single bed position, and patients are asked to hold their breath for up to 20 s. Statistical limitations are overcome by acquiring over multiple breath holds and summing the data.

7.3 4D PET/CT

4D CT has now been used for over a decade to assess tumour motion over the course of the respiratory cycle [9, 10]. A surrogate signal assumed to reflect respiration is acquired in parallel with CT data acquisition. Pressure sensors, strain-gauge belts, spirometry systems and optoelectronic systems have all been used to provide such a signal.

The CT acquisition may be either prospective or retrospective. In the prospective case, the signal is used to identify a specific part of the respiratory cycle and limit data acquisition to this window. Radiation doses are therefore of the same order of magnitude as for conventional CT imaging.

In the retrospective mode, data is acquired such that projection data are acquired over the entire respiratory cycle. Consequently such scans are characterised by a longer scan time and higher patient dose. Data can be binned according to either the relative amplitude or phase of the external signal (see Fig. 7.1).

The same external signal can be used to bin the PET data and reconstruct 4D PET images. As well enabling motion tracking, 4D PET also has the potential for improved spatial resolution and more accurate quantitation. As with breath-hold PET, respiratory gated PET images will suffer from reduced signal to noise unless imaging time is extended.

Ideally attenuation correction should be undertaken with a 4D CT dataset [11, 12], although this may not always be possible depending on the manufacturer. Particular care needs to be given to the synchronisation of the CT and PET images. For example, the amplitude-based binning illustrated in Fig. 7.1 would not provide a well-matched set of images if the PET data is binned according to phase. Even if phase binning was used in each case, the temporal resolution of the CT is determined by the tube rotation time and therefore the width of the gates will not necessarily be equivalent between the modalities.

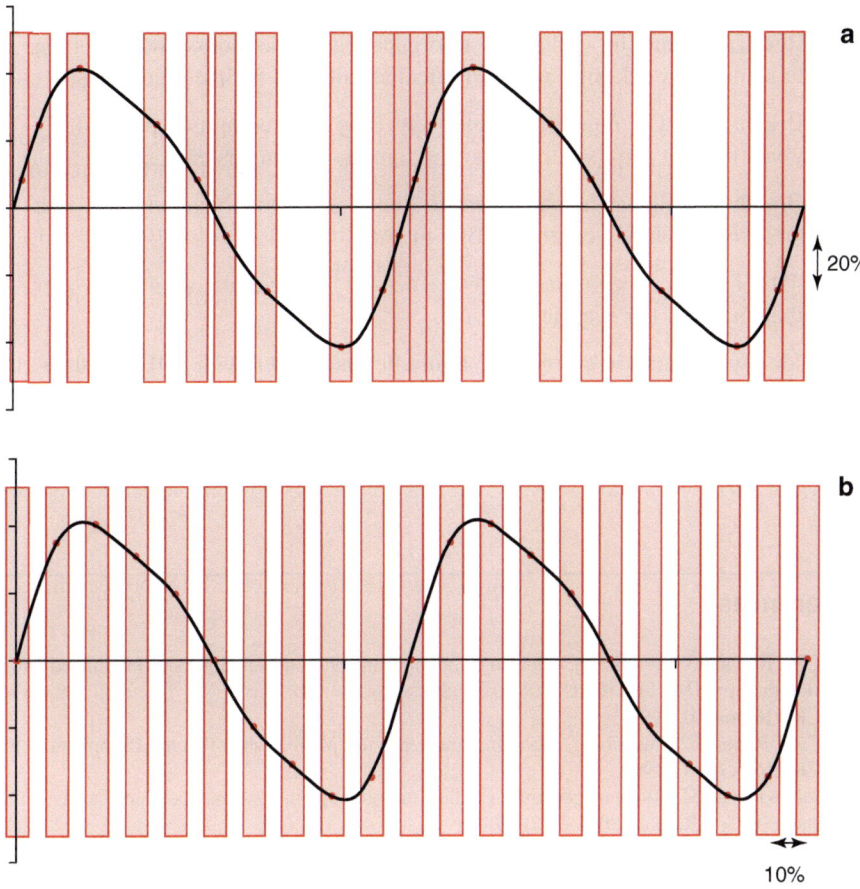

Fig. 7.1 Illustration of a respiratory surrogate signal from which gates have been derived using either (**a**) amplitude binning or (**b**) phase binning

Key Points

- The most important limiting factors affecting radiation delivery is the ability to match the positioning of the radiation beams to the target in question.

- To account for positioning uncertainties, the standard practice is to add a margin to the defined target.

- The addition of margins clearly reduces the therapeutic index (the relationship between the dose delivered to the tumour and the dose delivered to the surrounding tissue).

- Respiratory motion will affect all organs within the thorax and abdomen to some degree. Lungs are most affected followed by liver and breast.
- Breath-hold CT imaging is relatively easy to accomplish, particularly given the fast acquisition times which modern scanners can achieve.
- Breath holding can be patient controlled or alternatively undertaken with an active breathing control (ABC) method.
- 4D CT has now been used for over a decade to assess tumour motion over the course of the respiratory cycle.
- Ideally attenuation correction should be undertaken with a 4D CT dataset, although this may not always be possible depending on the manufacturer.
- Synchronisation of the CT and PET images is necessary.

References

1. ICRU Report 83: Prescribing, recording, and reporting photon-beam intensity-modulated radiation therapy (IMRT). J ICRU. 2010;10(1):NP.
2. ICRU Report 50. 1993.
3. ICRU Report 62 prescribing, recording and reporting photon beam therapy (Supplement to ICRU Report 50). 1999.
4. Cole AJ, et al. Motion management for radical radiotherapy in non-small cell lung cancer. Clin Oncol (R Coll Radiol). 2014;26(2):67–80.
5. Kawano T, Ohtake E, Inoue T. Deep-inspiration breath-hold PET/CT of lung cancer: maximum standardized uptake value analysis of 108 patients. J Nucl Med. 2008;49(8):1223–31.
6. Nehmeh SA, et al. Deep-inspiration breath-hold PET/CT of the thorax. J Nucl Med. 2007;48(1):22–6.
7. Shyn PB, et al. Minimizing image misregistration during PET/CT-guided percutaneous interventions with monitored breath-hold PET and CT acquisitions. J Vasc Interv Radiol. 2011;22(9):1287–92.
8. Torizuka T, et al. Single 20-second acquisition of deep-inspiration breath-hold PET/CT: clinical feasibility for lung cancer. J Nucl Med. 2009;50(10):1579–84.
9. Ford EC, et al. Respiration-correlated spiral CT: a method of measuring respiratory-induced anatomic motion for radiation treatment planning. Med Phys. 2003;30(1):88–97.
10. Vedam SS, et al. Acquiring a four-dimensional computed tomography dataset using an external respiratory signal. Phys Med Biol. 2003;48(1):45–62.
11. Sakaguchi Y, et al. Importance of gated CT acquisition for the quantitative improvement of the gated PET/CT in moving phantom. Ann Nucl Med. 2010;24(7):507–14.
12. Nagel CCA, et al. Phased attenuation correction in respiration correlated computed tomography/positron emitted tomography. Med Phys. 2006;33(6):1840–7.

Part III

PET/CT in Radiotherapy Planning - Current Evidence and Applications

Lung Cancer

8

Angus O'Connor and Helen M. Betts

Content

References.. 49

The most significant impact of PET/CT in lung cancer radiotherapy planning is through the well-established improvement in primary tumour staging compared with conventional CT alone. FDG (^{18}F-fluoro-deoxy-glucose) PET/CT has been shown to identify distant metastases in up to 30% of cases compared with conventional CT staging [1, 2]. Identification of tumour outside a potential radiotherapy field precludes radical treatment with curative intent which significantly changes patient management (Fig. 8.1). It may also identify occult lesions in critical anatomical sites such as the spine and weight bearing bones which require local treatment.

Maximum standardised uptake value (SUV_{max}) has been shown in some studies of both conventionally fractionated and stereotactic radiotherapy to be a predictor of progression-free survival, but the literature is by no means conclusive in this regard [3, 4]. In addition, there is no consensus on cutoff SUV values. Dose alteration on the basis of SUV_{max} has been suggested but convincing outcome data does not as yet exist. Pretreatment SUV analysis of lung tissue has also been shown in one study to identify patients at high risk of radiation pneumonitis [5].

A. O'Connor
Department of Radiology, Nottingham University Hospitals NHS Trust, Nottingham, UK
e-mail: Richard.O'Connor@nuh.nhs.uk

H.M. Betts
Department of Medical Physics and Clinical Engineering, Nottingham University Hospitals NHS Trust, Nottingham, UK
e-mail: Helen.Betts2@nuh.nhs.uk

© Springer International Publishing Switzerland 2017
S. Chua (ed.), *PET/CT in Radiotherapy Planning*, Clinicians' Guides to Radionuclide Hybrid Imaging - PET/CT, DOI 10.1007/978-3-319-54744-2_8

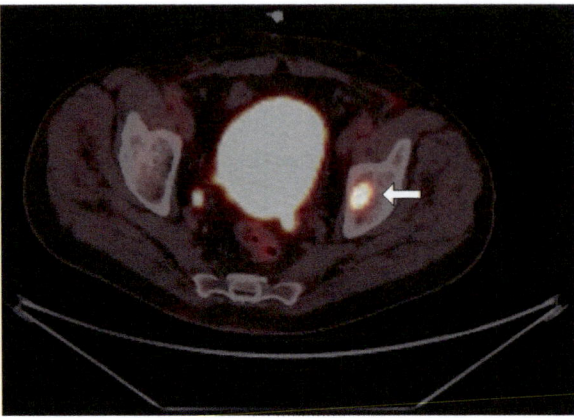

Fig. 8.1 Fused axial FDG-PET/CT scan in a 73-year-old male patient being assessed for radical radiotherapy treatment of a primary bronchogenic carcinoma. Image through the lower pelvis demonstrates focal increased activity in the left acetabulum (*arrow*) in keeping with a metastasis, precluding radical treatment with curative intent

Practical radiotherapy planning involves a compromise between dose escalation in the primary tumour, adequate coverage of involved nodal stations and minimising toxicity to normal structures. PET/CT may be used as a direct aid when delineating treatment volumes on a planning CT study. Justification for this is supported by the high negative predictive value of FDG-PET (>90%) in staging mediastinal lymph nodes [6], allowing the oncologist to restrict gross target volumes where possible. FDG-PET is also being widely used to reduce treatment portal size by distinguishing FDG-negative atelectasis from PET-positive primary tumour (Fig. 8.2). Although definitive outcome data to support this practice is limited, studies have demonstrated the accuracy of FDG-PET/CT in tumour volume delineation compared with pathological specimens [7]. PET/CT has also been shown to improve interobserver variability in delineating treatment volumes which is highly desirable though again unproven to lead to more favourable outcomes in itself.

Fusion of FDG-PET and planning CT images or dedicated PET/CT planning sessions is the logical next step and has been the subject of considerable interest. The principal challenges are reconciling the limited resolution of PET with the precise collimation of radiotherapy fields demanded for modern dose escalation and the problem of respiratory motion. At present the evidence would not appear to justify routine dedicated 3D FDG-PET/CT internal gross tumour volume planning compared with 4D contrast-enhanced CT which is the

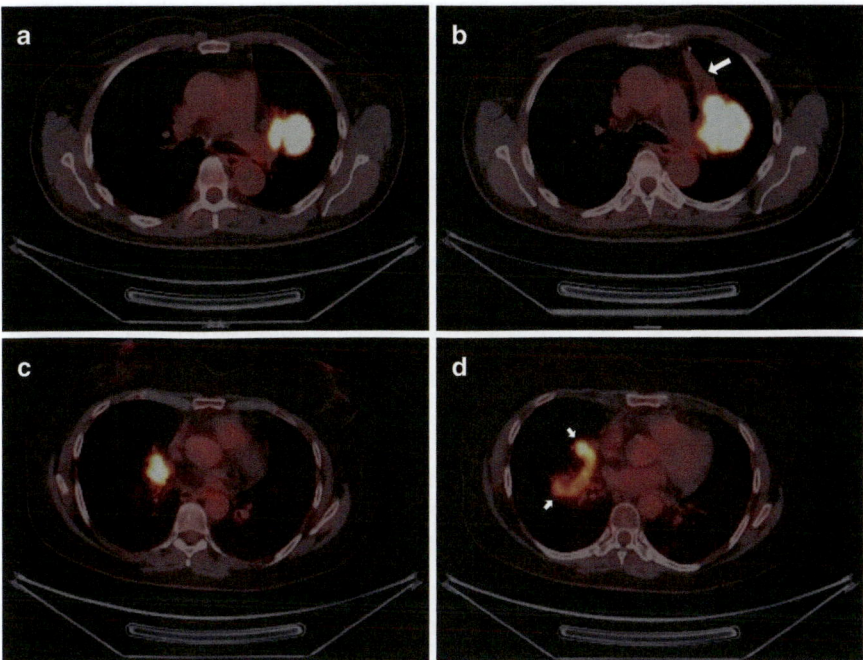

Fig. 8.2 Fused axial FDG-PET/CT images in patients with primary bronchogenic carcinoma being assessed for radical radiotherapy. (**a**) A 69-year-old male patient with a large left-sided tumour. (**b**) Inferiorly the metabolically active tumour can be clearly separated from adjacent atelectasis (*arrow*), allowing a reduction in target volume. (**c**) A 52-year-old female patient with increased activity in a right-sided central tumour. (**d**) Increased activity is seen distally anteriorly and laterally in wedge-shaped portions of tissue contiguous with the tumour (*arrows*). Due to the increased activity in this area, it is not possible to accurately separate atelectasis and consolidation from tumour making precise radiotherapy planning difficult

current gold standard [8]. 4D PET/CT radiotherapy planning may lead to improved target volume definition but is not yet widely available.

Hypoxia has long been known to cause resistance to radiotherapy. Selective PET tracers which accumulate in hypoxic tissues have therefore generated considerable research interest [9] (Fig. 8.3). Comparisons with FDG images show that regions of hypoxia do not necessarily correlate with the areas of the highest metabolic activity, demonstrating that FDG is not a reliable surrogate marker for hypoxia [10]. Future trials are likely to focus on whether hypoxia PET scans can identify the patients who would benefit from dose modulation in hypoxic regions.

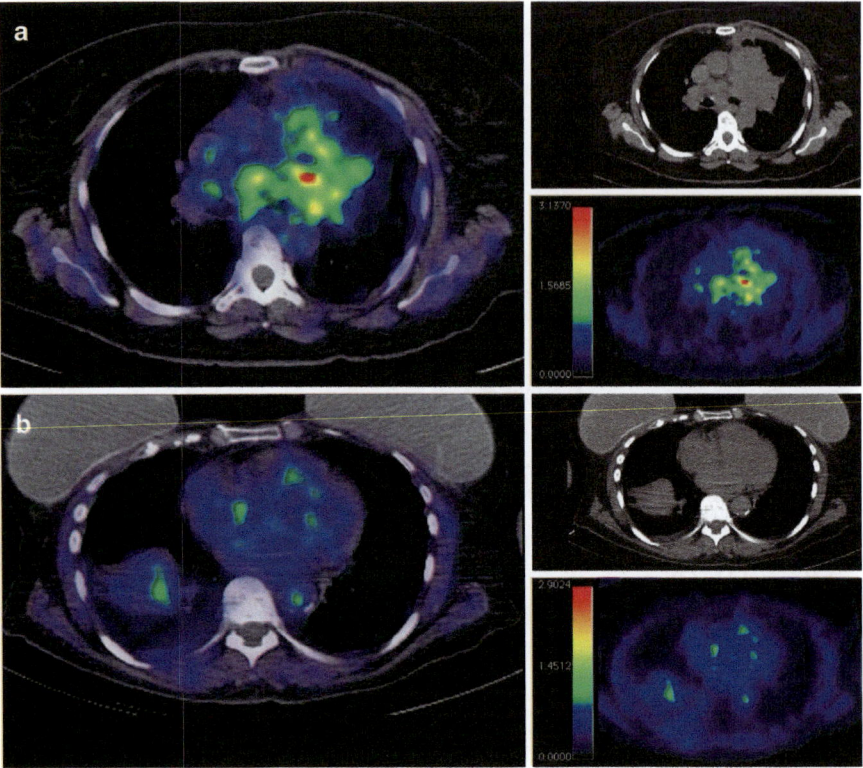

Fig. 8.3 Fused PET/CT images of primary bronchogenic carcinoma with HX4, a promising hypoxia imaging tracer. (**a**) Markedly increased activity is seen in a left-sided tumour extending into subcarinal lymphadenopathy indicating hypoxia and possible radiotherapy resistance. (**b**) In another patient, activity in the right lower lobe lesion is similar to background suggesting the absence of generalised tumour hypoxia *(Images courtesy of Threshold pharmaceuticals)*

Key Points

- Impact of PET/CT in lung cancer radiotherapy planning is through the well-established improvement in primary tumour staging compared with conventional CT alone.
- 18F-FDG-PET/CT has been shown to identify distant metastases in up to 30% of cases compared with conventional CT staging.
- Identification of tumour outside a potential radiotherapy field precludes radical treatment with curative intent which significantly changes patient management.

- It may also identify occult lesions in critical anatomical sites such as the spine and weight bearing bones which require local treatment.
- Maximum standardised uptake value (SUV_{max}) has been shown in some studies of both conventionally fractionated and stereotactic radiotherapy to be a predictor of progression-free survival, but the literature is by no means conclusive in this regard.
- There is no consensus on cutoff SUV values. Dose alteration on the basis of SUV_{max} has been suggested, but convincing outcome data does not as yet exist.
- PET/CT may be used as a direct aid when delineating treatment volumes on a planning CT study particularly through the high negative predictive value in mediastinal lymph node evaluation.
- FDG-PET is also being widely used to reduce treatment portal size by distinguishing FDG-negative atelectasis from PET-positive primary tumour.
- 4D PET/CT radiotherapy planning may lead to improved target volume definition but is not yet widely available.
- Hypoxia has long been known to cause resistance to radiotherapy. Selective PET tracers which accumulate in hypoxic tissues provide complimentary information to FDG imaging, possibly in the future guiding dose escalation strategies.

References

1. Abramyuk A, Appold S, Zöphel K, Hietschold V, Baumann M, Abolmaali N. Quantitative modifications of TNM staging, clinical staging and therapeutic intent by FDG-PET/CT in patients with non-small cell lung cancer scheduled for radiotherapy—a retrospective study. Lung Cancer. 2012;78(2):148–52.
2. Mac Manus MP. Use of PET/CT for staging and radiation therapy planning in patients with non-small cell lung cancer. Q J Nucl Med Mol Imaging. 2010;54(5):510–20.
3. Ulger S, Demirci NY, Eroglu FN, Cengiz HH, Tunc M, Tatci E, Yilmaz U, Cetin E, Avci E, Cengiz M. High FDG uptake predicts poorer survival in locally advanced nonsmall cell lung cancer patients undergoing curative radiotherapy, independently of tumor size. J Cancer Res Clin Oncol. 2014;140(3):495–502.
4. Lin MY, Wu M, Brennan S, Campeau MP, Binns DS, MacManus M, Solomon B, Hicks RJ, Fisher RJ, Ball DL. Absence of a relationship between tumor ^{18}F-fluorodeoxyglucose standardized uptake value and survival in patients treated with definitive radiotherapy for non-small-cell lung cancer. J Thorac Oncol. 2014;9(3):377–82.
5. Castillo R, Pham N, Ansari S, Meshkov D, Castillo S, Li M, Olanrewaju A, Hobbs B, Castillo E, Guerrero T. Pre-radiotherapy FDG PET predicts radiation pneumonitis in lung cancer. Radiat Oncol. 2014;9:74.

6. Darling GE, Maziak DE, Inculet RI, Gulenchyn KY, Driedger AA, Ung YC, Gu CS, Kuruvilla MS, Cline KJ, Julian JA, Evans WK, Levine MN. Positron emission tomography-computed tomography compared with invasive mediastinal staging in non-small cell lung cancer: results of mediastinal staging in the early lung positron emission tomography trial. J Thorac Oncol. 2011;6(8):1367–72.
7. Yu HM, Liu YF, Hou M, Liu J, Li XN, Yu JM. Evaluation of gross tumor size using CT, 18F-FDG PET, integrated ^{18}F-FDG PET/CT and pathological analysis in non-small cell lung cancer. Eur J Radiol. 2009;72(1):104–13. doi:10.1016/j.ejrad.2008.06.015.
8. Duan YL, Li JB, Zhang YJ, Wang W, Li FX, Sun XR, Guo YL, Shang DP. Comparison of primary target volumes delineated on four-dimensional CT and ^{18}F-FDG PET/CT of non-small-cell lung cancer. Radiat Oncol. 2014;9:182. doi:10.1186/1748-717X-9-182.
9. Horsman MR, Mortensen LS, Petersen JB, Busk M, Overgaard J. Imaging hypoxia to improve radiotherapy outcome. Nat Rev Clin Oncol. 2012;9(12):674–87.
10. Cherk MH, Foo SS, Poon AM, Knight SR, Murone C, Papenfuss AT, Sachinidis JI, Saunder TH, O'Keefe GJ, Scott AM. Lack of correlation of hypoxic cell fraction and angiogenesis with glucose metabolic rate in non-small cell lung cancer assessed by ^{18}F-Fluoromisonidazole and 18F-FDG PET. J Nucl Med. 2006;47(12):1921–6.

Head and Neck Cancers

9

Liam Welsh and Kate Newbold

Contents

9.1　Introduction... 51
9.2　Staging... 51
9.3　Target Volume Definition...................................... 52
9.4　Dose Painting and Adaptive Radiotherapy........ 53
9.5　Treatment Response Evaluation 54
References.. 54

9.1　Introduction

Clinical practice in treating head and neck cancers (HNC) makes use of ^{18}F-fluorodeoxyglucose (FDG) PET/CT, but other tracers are under investigation and may provide additional clinically useful information [1].

9.2　Staging

Radiotherapy (RT) planning for HNC relies on accurate and anatomically precise staging information. The UK Intercollegiate Standing Committee on Nuclear Medicine 2013 recognises the following indications for FDG-PET/CT staging of HNC: equivocal clinical staging, patients at high risk of disseminated disease and identification of occult primary tumour(s) in patients presenting with metastatic squamous cell carcinoma in cervical lymph nodes (LN). Whilst systematic reviews show FDG-PET/CT to be highly accurate in diagnosing and staging HNC [2, 3], FDG-PET/CT scanning lacks sensitivity for LNs <5 mm, necrotic LNs and tumours with low metabolic activity.

L. Welsh, MA PhD MRCP FRCR (✉) • K. Newbold, MD MRCP FRCR
Head and Neck Unit, Royal Marsden NHS Foundation Trust, London, UK
e-mail: Liam.Welsh@rmh.nhs.uk

© Springer International Publishing Switzerland 2017
S. Chua (ed.), *PET/CT in Radiotherapy Planning*, Clinicians' Guides
to Radionuclide Hybrid Imaging - PET/CT, DOI 10.1007/978-3-319-54744-2_9

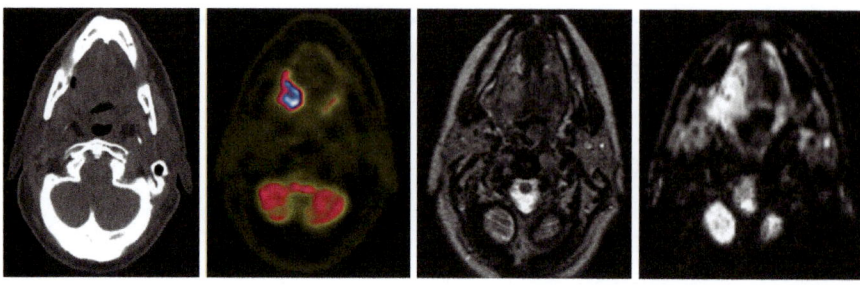

Fig. 9.1 Multimodality functional imaging from a patient with a T3N2bM0 HPV-positive squamous cell carcinoma of the right oropharynx. All images were obtained using identical patient positioning and thermoplastic mask immobilisation before starting radical chemo-RT. Equivalent axial slices are shown at the level of the primary tumour. *From the left*: CT, ^{18}F-FDG-PET, T2w MRI and diffusion-weighted MRI (Courtesy of Dr. Alex Dunlop)

Table 9.1 Summary of strengths and weaknesses of FDG-PET/CT for radiotherapy planning for head and neck cancer

Advantages
Reduced interobserver variation in GTV delineation
Reduced size of GTV
Identifying tumour or LN missed by CT/MRI
Identifying GTV regions potentially requiring additional radiation dose
Disadvantages
Limited spatial resolution
Lack of standardised method for signal segmentation
False-positive PET readings due to inflammation/biopsy

9.3 Target Volume Definition

Consensus guidelines have standardised LN delineation for HNC RT planning, but not the delineation of primary HNC tumours. Since the introduction of intensity-modulated RT (IMRT) for HNC, there has been a shift from anatomically based primary clinical target volumes (CTV) to volumetric primary CTVs based on marginal expansion from a primary gross tumour volume (GTV). The volumetric CTV approach has greater dependency on accurate imaging data, and in this context FDG-PET/CT may be particularly valuable. Correlation of surgical specimens with pre-operative imaging shows that FDG-PET/CT-defined GTVs are closer to those defined by histology than either CT or MRI [4]. However, techniques for delineating GTVs using FDG-PET/CT have not been standardised, and there is no consensus on the optimal methodology [1]. Currently, the best approach is to incorporate data from all available imaging modalities (Fig. 9.1), along with clinical findings, into HNC GTV definition [5]. Strengths and weaknesses of FDG-PET/CT for HNC RT planning are summarised in Table 9.1.

9 Head and Neck Cancers

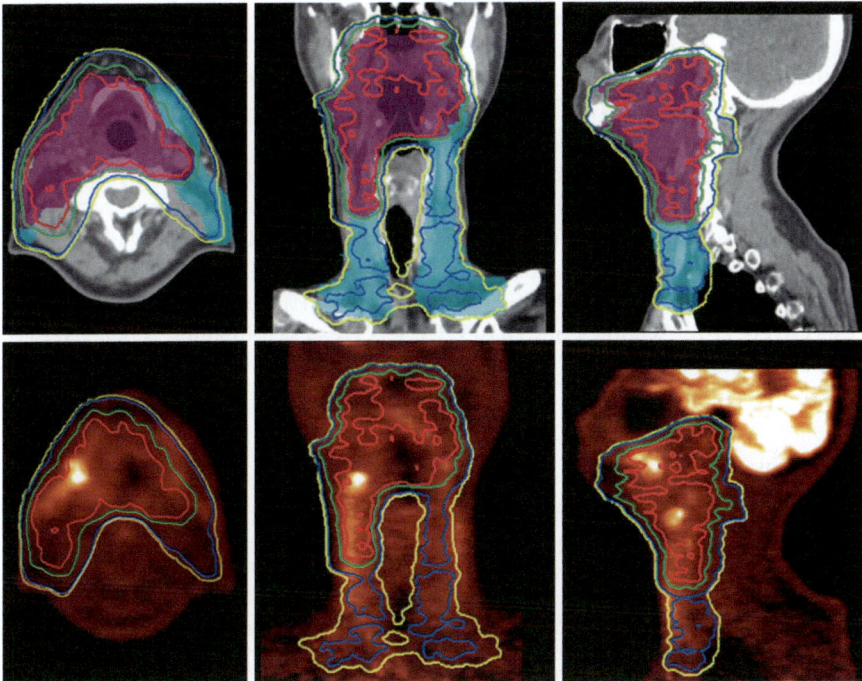

Fig. 9.2 Planned radical radiotherapy dose distribution, for the same patient shown in Fig. 9.1, overlaid on the RT planning CT (*top*) and pretreatment ^{18}F-FDG-PET (*bottom*). *The pink and blue colour washes* on *the top panel* denoted the high- (PTV1) and low- (PTV2) dose PTVs, respectively. *Coloured contours* on both panels denote radiotherapy isodose levels: *red* 100% prescription dose PTV1 (65.0 Gy), *green* 95% prescription dose PTV1 (61.7 Gy), *blue* 100% prescription dose PTV2 (54.0 Gy) and *yellow* 95% prescription dose PTV2 (51.3 Gy). The heterogeneity of FDG uptake within PTV1 is evident, naturally lending itself to IMRT dose painting (Courtesy of Dr. Alex Dunlop)

9.4 Dose Painting and Adaptive Radiotherapy

FDG-PET/CT may identify tumour subvolumes for IMRT dose boosting, as can be appreciated from Fig. 9.2. A phase 1 study of FDG-PET/CT-based GTV subvolume dose escalation has demonstrated the clinical feasibility of this approach [6].

Adaptive IMRT modifies an IMRT plan according to changes in GTV and/or surrounding normal tissues on serial CT imaging through the course of treatment. Adaptive IMRT for HNC may improve delivered RT doses relative to conventional IMRT. It is not yet clear whether FDG-PET/CT adds significant additional information to CT alone for adaptive IMRT, and so far one comparative study has found no benefit from the addition of FDG-PET/CT data [7].

9.5 Treatment Response Evaluation

Pretreatment FDG-PET/CT can identify patients at high risk of treatment failure [8]. Sequential FDG-PET/CT imaging through a course of radical RT may provide data with greater predictive power [9].

After primary radical chemo-RT for HNC, imaging is used to assess response. In a meta-analysis, the weighted mean (95% CI) pooled estimates for sensitivity, specificity, positive predictive value and negative predictive value of FDG-PET/CT for detection of residual disease following radical chemo-RT for HNC were 87.7% (83.4–91.2%), 87.8% (85.1–90.2%), 75.7% (70.8–80.1%) and 94.3% (92.2–96.0%), respectively [10]. Accuracy of FDG-PET/CT is greatest if imaging is delayed until ≥ 12 weeks after RT [10].

> **Key Points**
>
> - Radiotherapy (RT) planning for HNC relies on accurate and anatomically precise staging information.
> - Consensus guidelines have standardised LN delineation for HNC RT planning, but not the delineation of primary HNC tumours.
> - Introduction of intensity-modulated RT (IMRT) for HNC led to a shift from anatomically based primary clinical target volumes (CTV) to volumetric primary CTVs based on marginal expansion from a primary gross tumour volume (GTV).
> - FDG-PET/CT may identify tumour subvolumes for IMRT dose boosting.
> - Pretreatment FDG-PET/CT can identify patients at high risk of treatment failure.
> - Sequential FDG-PET/CT imaging through a course of radical RT may provide data with greater predictive power.
> - After primary radical chemo-RT for HNC, imaging is used to assess response. Accuracy of FDG-PET/CT is greatest if imaging is delayed until ≥ 12 weeks after RT.

References

1. Newbold K, Powell C. PET/CT in radiotherapy planning for head and neck cancer. Front Oncol. 2012;2:189.
2. Evangelista L, Cervino AR, Chondrogiannis S, Marzola MC, Maffione AM, Colletti PM, Muzzio PC, Rubello D. Comparison between anatomical cross-sectional imaging and 18F-FDG PET/CT in the staging, restaging, treatment response, and long-term surveillance of

squamous cell head and neck cancer: a systematic literature overview. Nucl Med Commun. 2014;35:123–34.
3. Rohde M, Dyrvig A-K, Johansen J, Sørensen JA, Gerke O, Nielsen AL, Høilund-Carlsen PF, Godballe C. 18F-fluoro-deoxy-glucose-positron emission tomography/computed tomography in diagnosis of head and neck squamous cell carcinoma: a systematic review and meta-analysis. Eur J Cancer. 2014;50:2271–9.
4. Caldas-Magalhaes J, Kasperts N, Kooij N, van den Berg CAT, Terhaard CHJ, Raaijmakers CPJ, Philippens MEP. Validation of imaging with pathology in laryngeal cancer: accuracy of the registration methodology. Int J Radiat Oncol Biol Phys. 2012;82:e289–98.
5. Thiagarajan A, Caria N, Schöder H, Iyer NG, Wolden S, Wong RJ, Sherman E, Fury MG, Lee N. Target volume delineation in oropharyngeal cancer: impact of PET, MRI, and physical examination. Int J Radiat Oncol Biol Phys. 2012;83:220–7.
6. Madani I, Duthoy W, Derie C, de Gersem W, Boterberg T, Saerens M, Jacobs F, Grégoire V, Lonneux M, Vakaet L, Vanderstraeten B, Bauters W, Bonte K, Thierens H, de Neve W. Positron emission tomography-guided, focal-dose escalation using intensity-modulated radiotherapy for head and neck cancer. Int J Radiat Oncol Biol Phys. 2007;68:126–35.
7. Castadot P, Geets X, Lee JA, Grégoire V. Adaptive functional image-guided IMRT in pharyngo-laryngeal squamous cell carcinoma: is the gain in dose distribution worth the effort? Radiother Oncol. 2011;101:343–50.
8. Due AK, Vogelius IR, Aznar MC, Bentzen SM, Berthelsen AK, Korreman SS, Loft A, Kristensen CA, Specht L. Recurrences after intensity modulated radiotherapy for head and neck squamous cell carcinoma more likely to originate from regions with high baseline [18F]-FDG uptake. Radiother Oncol. 2014;111:360–5.
9. Powell C, Schmidt M, Borri M, Koh D-M, Partridge M, Riddell A, Cook G, Bhide SA, Nutting CM, Harrington KJ, Newbold KL. Changes in functional imaging parameters following induction chemotherapy have important implications for individualised patient-based treatment regimens for advanced head and neck cancer. Radiother Oncol. 2013;106:112–7.
10. Gupta T, Master Z, Kannan S, Agarwal JP, Ghsoh-Laskar S, Rangarajan V, Murthy V, Budrukkar A. Diagnostic performance of post-treatment FDG PET or FDG PET/CT imaging in head and neck cancer: a systematic review and meta-analysis. Eur J Nucl Med Mol Imaging. 2011;38:2083–95.

GI Malignancy

10

Irene Chong and Diana Tait

Contents

10.1 Introduction 57
10.2 Rectal Cancer 57
10.3 Oesophageal and Pancreatic Cancer 59
10.4 Summary 60
References 61

10.1 Introduction

GI malignancy covers four main tumour sites: oesophagogastric, hepatobiliary, colorectal and anus with radiotherapy having an important role to play in each of these sites. PET/CT is not standard in the planning procedure for these patients, but research is ongoing and most available data relates to rectal cancer [1, 2].

10.2 Rectal Cancer

The potential benefits of PET scanning in rectal RT planning are illustrated by a study comparing CT-PET-, MR-PET- and FDG-PET-based tumour length measurements with pathology in patients receiving short-course RT (5×5 Gy) and surgery [3]. Although no significant correlation was found between CT-based measurements with the resection specimen, a modest correlation was detected with MR-based measurements (Pearson's correlation = 0.55, $p < 0.001$), and a good correlation was confirmed

I. Chong (✉) • D. Tait
Clinical Oncology, The Royal Marsden NHS Foundation Trust and The Institute of Cancer Research, London, UK
e-mail: Irene.chong@icr.ac.uk

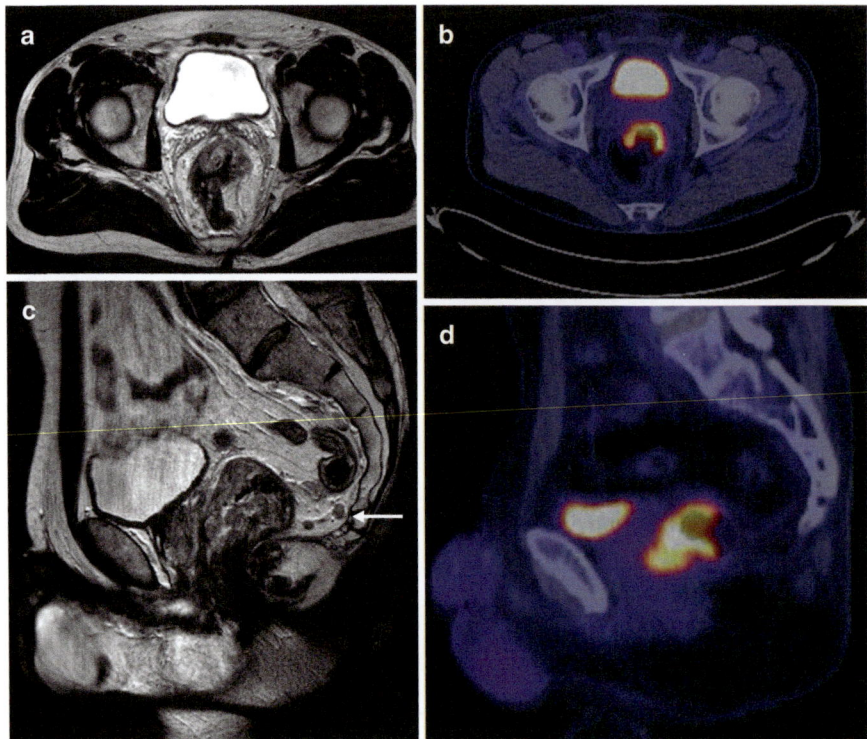

Fig. 10.1 MRI and 18F-fluorodeoxyglucose positron emission tomography (FDG-PET) images of a patient with locally advanced rectal cancer prior to chemoradiotherapy. The rectal tumour is demonstrated as an annular mass on axial MRI imaging (**a**). The most metabolically active part of the tumour extends from the 10 to 4 o'clock position where it abuts the prostate and seminal vesicles (**b**). Enlarged lymph nodes with mixed signal and irregular borders are observed on MRI (**c**—*white arrow*). However, these lymph nodes were of low FDG avidity and were not reliably detected by PET (**d**), emphasising the importance of using MRI in conjunction with PET for RT planning

with manual FDG-PET measurements (Pearson's correlation = 0.72, $p < 0.001$), but the best correlation with pathology was observed with automatic PET/CT based measurements (Pearson correlation = 0.91, $p < 0.001$). An overestimation of the rectal tumour diameter and volume using manual MRI-based measurements compared with PET-based contouring has also been reported [4]. This is an important consideration, especially for low rectal cancers where the caudal border of the treatment volume may be tailored, resulting in avoidance of sphincter irradiation (Fig. 10.1).

The use of FDG-PET/CT has been shown to reduce the interobserver variability in rectal tumour delineation. In a recent study, GTVs generated from automatic contours on PET scan were compared with GTVs manually delineated by multiple observers [2]. GTVs based on PET were more consistent with the PET auto-contouring method. Moreover, the CTV based on PET extended outside of the CTV used in clinical practice in almost a third of patients, suggesting that the integration of PET in the RT planning process in rectal cancer has the potential to avoid geographical misses. This may have important clinical implications for defining the phase II 'boost' for rectal tumours with involved circumferential resection margins [5].

10.3 Oesophageal and Pancreatic Cancer

Radiotherapy planning for oesophagogastric carcinomas is notoriously difficult because of poor tumour delineation on standard imaging. CT demonstrates bulk disease but has limitations in defining longitudinal spread of disease, and endoscopy only gives the luminal dimensions. FDG-PET has been observed to improve intra- and interobserver variability. Using endoscopic ultrasound (EUS) as gold standard, FDG-PET facilitated a more accurate delineation of oesophageal tumour length compared with CT [6]. In pancreatic cancer, the use of FDG-PET fusion with planning CT has resulted in GTVs that were smaller overall compared with CT alone [7] (Figs. 10.2 and 10.3).

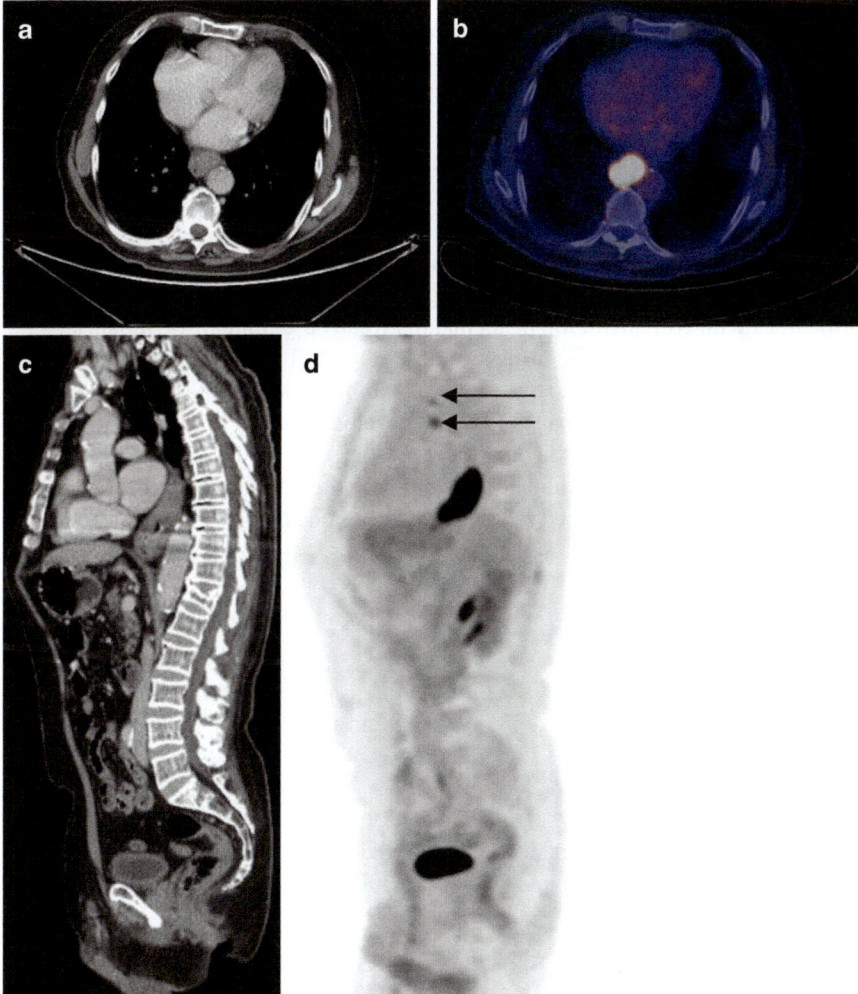

Fig. 10.2 CT and 18F-fluorodeoxyglucose positron emission tomography (FDG-PET) images of a patient with oesophageal cancer prior to chemoradiotherapy. The primary tumour is demonstrated as an annular mass on both CT and CT-PET (**a** and **b**). Metabolically active hilar lymph nodes are present on PET/CT (**d**—*black arrows*). Lymph node spread was not detected on cross-sectional CT

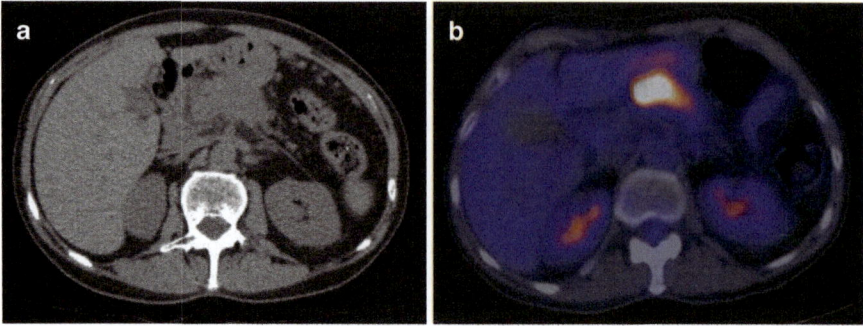

Fig. 10.3 CT and 18F-fluorodeoxyglucose positron emission tomography (FDG-PET) images of a patient with locally advanced pancreatic cancer prior to chemo-RT. A poorly enhancing mass is seen in the body of the pancreas with evidence of vascular encasement (**a**). FDG avidity is observed to correspond with the mass at the junction between the body and tail of the pancreas (**b**)

10.4 Summary

In the format that's available to most clinicians at the present time, PET has significant limitations for radiotherapy planning [8]. Patient position, slice thickness and difficulties with co-registration mean that there can be an unrealistic reliance on the imaging available to our diagnostic systems. FDG-PET can be unreliable in distinguishing between benign and pathological lymph nodes because of non-specific FDG uptake within macrophages [9]. The development of PET tracers measuring cell proliferation and hypoxia has the potential to improve tumour specificity. Further work is required to validate their utility in the RT planning process, particularly in the setting of advanced radiotherapy techniques [10].

Key Points

- In GI malignancy, PET/CT is not standard in the planning procedure for these patients, but research is ongoing and most available data relates to rectal cancer.

Rectal Cancer

- An overestimation of the rectal tumour diameter and volume using manual MRI-based measurements compared with PET-based contouring has also been reported.
- FDG-PET/CT has been shown to reduce the interobserver variability in rectal tumour delineation.

- Integration of PET in the RT planning process in rectal cancer has the potential to avoid geographical misses.

Oesophageal Cancer

- Radiotherapy planning for oesophagogastric carcinomas is notoriously difficult because of poor tumour delineation on standard imaging.
- FDG-PET has been observed to improve intra- and interobserver variability.
- Using endoscopic ultrasound (EUS) as gold standard, FDG-PET facilitated a more accurate delineation of oesophageal tumour length compared with CT.

Pancreatic Cancer

- FDG-PET fusion with planning CT has resulted in GTVs that were smaller overall compared with CT alone.

References

1. Krengli M, et al. Target volume delineation for preoperative radiotherapy of rectal cancer: inter-observer variability and potential impact of FDG-PET/CT imaging. Technol Cancer Res Treat. 2010;9(4):393–8.
2. Buijsen J, et al. FDG-PET-CT reduces the interobserver variability in rectal tumor delineation. Radiother Oncol. 2012;102(3):371–6.
3. Buijsen J, et al. FDG-PET provides the best correlation with the tumor specimen compared to MRI and CT in rectal cancer. Radiother Oncol. 2011;98(2):270–6.
4. Braendengen M, et al. Delineation of gross tumor volume (GTV) for radiation treatment planning of locally advanced rectal cancer using information from MRI or FDG-PET/CT: a prospective study. Int J Radiat Oncol Biol Phys. 2011;81(4):e439–45.
5. Seierstad T, et al. MR-guided simultaneous integrated boost in preoperative radiotherapy of locally advanced rectal cancer following neoadjuvant chemotherapy. Radiother Oncol. 2009;93(2):279–84.
6. Konski A, et al. The integration of 18-fluoro-deoxy-glucose positron emission tomography and endoscopic ultrasound in the treatment-planning process for esophageal carcinoma. Int J Radiat Oncol Biol Phys. 2005;61(4):1123–8.
7. Dalah E, et al. Variability of target and normal structure delineation using multimodality imaging for radiation therapy of pancreatic cancer. Int J Radiat Oncol Biol Phys. 2014;89(3):633–40.
8. MacManus M, et al. Use of PET and PET/CT for radiation therapy planning: IAEA expert report 2006–2007. Radiother Oncol. 2009;91(1):85–94.
9. Kantorova I, et al. Routine (18)F-FDG PET preoperative staging of colorectal cancer: comparison with conventional staging and its impact on treatment decision making. J Nucl Med. 2003;44(11):1784–8.
10. Roels S, et al. Biological image-guided radiotherapy in rectal cancer: is there a role for FMISO or FLT, next to FDG? Acta Oncol. 2008;47(7):1237–48.

Prostate Cancer

11

Daniel R. Henderson and Nicholas van As

Contents

11.1 Patient Selection for Treatment 63
11.2 Target Volume Delineation 64
References 65

The use of choline-PET/CT (C-PET/CT) in prostate radiotherapy planning has been evaluated in two principal settings: patient selection for treatment and target volume delineation. Choline-based tracers are used, as the relatively low glucose metabolism of prostate cancer means FDG-based tracers perform poorly [1].

11.1 Patient Selection for Treatment

Accurate staging is essential prior to radical radiotherapy treatment. The finding of lymph node or bone involvement may require a change in the radiotherapy field shape or make radiotherapy treatment inappropriate [2]. Evangelista et al. performed a meta-analysis of ten studies of C-PET/CT in intermediate- and high-risk localised prostate cancer prior to radical treatment [3]. They reported sensitivity of 49% and specificity of 95% for detection of lymph node metastases. In another meta-analysis, Umbehr et al. reported sensitivity and specificity of 84% and 79%, respectively [4]. Regarding bone metastases, similar accuracy to MRI has been reported [2]. These studies all concluded that there was insufficient evidence for the routine use of C-PET/CT in this setting. However, the use of C-PET/CT can be

D.R. Henderson • N. van As (✉)
Clinical Oncology, The Royal Marsden NHS Foundation Trust, London, UK
e-mail: Nicholas.VanAs@rmh.nhs.uk

Table 11.1 Percentage of positive choline-PET/CT scans for a given PSA level in patients with biochemical relapse

PSA level (ng/ml)	Percentage of positive scans (%)
0.2–1.0	19
1.0–3.0	46
>3.0	82

considered in patients at high risk of distant metastases with negative findings on conventional imaging such as MRI and bone scan.

In the setting of biochemical (PSA) failure following radical treatment, the site and extent of relapse determine further management [2]. Local recurrence following surgery may be treated with salvage radiotherapy. Oligometastatic disease may be treated with stereotactic radiotherapy [5] and more widespread disease with systemic therapy. A meta-analysis of 12 studies has demonstrated sensitivity and specificity of 85% and 88%, respectively, for detecting location(s) of relapse [4]. The use of C-PET/CT in this setting has been reported to change management in approximately 30% of cases [6, 7]. The ability to detect metastatic disease with a PSA under 20 ng/ml is a significant advantage over conventional imaging (CT or bone scan) [2]. However, it is important to select patients appropriately, as those with a PSA less than 1 ng/ml are unlikely to have a positive scan (see Table 11.1) [2]. To summarise, there is good evidence to support the use of C-PET/CT restaging following biochemical failure if further radiotherapy is being considered and PSA is above 1 ng/ml.

11.2 Target Volume Delineation

Due to its limited spatial resolution of around 5 mm, C-PET/CT has not been extensively evaluated for volume delineation [2]. However, C-PET/CT has been assessed for delineation of dominant intra-prostatic lesions (DIL). Increasing whole-prostate radiotherapy dose improves biochemical control but is limited by toxicity to surrounding organs. As the predominant site of intra-prostatic relapse is the DIL, it has been hypothesised that a radiotherapy boost to this area would improve disease control [8]. This approach requires an accurate method of delineating the DIL. Magnetic resonance imaging (MRI) has been the main technique used in clinical studies [9]. Van den Bergh et al. investigated whether C-PET/CT improved the accuracy of DIL delineation when added to MRI [10]. Pathology was used as the gold standard. They found only minimal improvement in accuracy and concluded that there was limited value for C-PET/CT in this setting. In summary, there is insufficient evidence to support the use of C-PET/CT in target volume delineation at present.

Key Points

- The use of choline-PET/CT (C-PET/CT) in prostate radiotherapy planning has been evaluated in two principal settings: patient selection for treatment and target volume delineation.

- Choline-based tracers are used, as the relatively low glucose metabolism of prostate cancer means FDG-based tracers perform poorly.
- Accurate staging is essential prior to radical radiotherapy treatment.
- The finding of lymph node or bone involvement may require a change in the radiotherapy field shape or make radiotherapy treatment inappropriate.
- There is good evidence to support the use of C-PET/CT restaging following biochemical failure if further radiotherapy is being considered and PSA is above 1 ng/ml.
- Due to its limited spatial resolution of around 5 mm, C-PET/CT has not been extensively evaluated for volume delineation.
- C-PET/CT has been assessed for delineation of dominant intra-prostatic lesions (DIL).
- There is insufficient evidence to support the use of C-PET/CT in target volume delineation at present.

References

1. Jadvar H. Imaging evaluation of prostate cancer with 18F-fluorodeoxyglucose PET/CT: utility and limitations. Eur J Nucl Med Mol Imaging. 2013;40(Suppl 1):S5–10.
2. Picchio M, Briganti A, Fanti S, Heidenreich A, Krause BJ, Messa C, et al. The role of choline positron emission tomography/computed tomography in the management of patients with prostate-specific antigen progression after radical treatment of prostate cancer. Eur Urol. 2011;59(1):51–60.
3. Evangelista L, Guttilla A, Zattoni F, Muzzio PC. Utility of choline positron emission tomography/computed tomography for lymph node involvement identification in intermediate- to high-risk prostate cancer: a systematic literature review and meta-analysis. Eur Urol. 2013;63(6):1040–8.
4. Umbehr MH, Muntener M, Hany T, Sulser T, Bachmann LM. The role of 11C-choline and 18F-fluorocholine positron emission tomography (PET) and PET/CT in prostate cancer: a systematic review and meta-analysis. Eur Urol. 2013;64(1):106–17.
5. Decaestecker K, De Meerleer G, Lambert B, Delrue L, Fonteyne V, Claeys T, et al. Repeated stereotactic body radiotherapy for oligometastatic prostate cancer recurrence. Radiat Oncol. 2014;9:135.
6. Jereczek-Fossa BA, Rodari M, Bonora M, Fanti P, Fodor C, Pepe G, et al. [11C]choline PET/CT impacts treatment decision making in patients with prostate cancer referred for radiotherapy. Clin Genitourin Cancer. 2014;12(3):155–9.
7. Souvatzoglou M, Krause BJ, Purschel A, Thamm R, Schuster T, Buck AK, et al. Influence of (11)C-choline PET/CT on the treatment planning for salvage radiation therapy in patients with biochemical recurrence of prostate cancer. Radiother Oncol. 2011;99(2):193–200.
8. Tree A, Jones C, Sohaib A, Khoo V, van As N. Prostate stereotactic body radiotherapy with simultaneous integrated boost: which is the best planning method? Radiat Oncol. 2013;8(1):228.

9. Fonteyne V, Villeirs G, Speleers B, De Neve W, De Wagter C, Lumen N, et al. Intensity-modulated radiotherapy as primary therapy for prostate cancer: report on acute toxicity after dose escalation with simultaneous integrated boost to intraprostatic lesion. Int J Radiat Oncol Biol Phys. 2008;72(3):799–807.
10. Van den Bergh L, Koole M, Isebaert S, Joniau S, Deroose CM, Oyen R, et al. Is there an additional value of (1)(1)C-choline PET-CT to T2-weighted MRI images in the localization of intraprostatic tumor nodules? Int J Radiat Oncol Biol Phys. 2012;83(5):1486–92.

Gynaecological Cancers

12

Susan Lalondrelle

Contents

12.1 Cervix Cancer 67
12.2 Endometrial Cancer. 70
12.3 Novel PET Tracers 70
References. 71

12.1 Cervix Cancer

^{18}FDG PET/CT is routinely used in the staging of primary cervix cancer for assessment of nodal involvement and distant metastasis (Fig. 12.1). A sensitivity and specificity of 83% and 95%, respectively, has been shown for detecting pelvic lymph node metastasis [1]. Whilst the sensitivity and specificity for para-aortic microscopic nodal disease is inferior, PET/CT has been incorporated into the radiotherapy planning process, primarily as an aid to defining nodal disease for dose escalation but also for GTV definition.

PET/CT-based GTV delineation has been compared to MRI both to define the superior border of pelvic/ para-aortic fields and in defining the primary target. The optimum SUVmax threshold for delineation is a subject of ongoing studies. Upasani et al. [2] have described a 30% SUVmax to have the best correlation with MRI-based primary tumour volume; others have utilised an SUVmax of 40% [3].

The main use of PET/CT in cervix radiotherapy planning has been the identification of lymph node targets for boosting dose (Fig. 12.2). Grigsby et al. [4] have reported 208 patients safely escalating dose to PET-positive pelvic lymph nodes 2–3 cm in size to 69.4 Gy, >3 cm to 74.1 Gy, using a concomitant IMRT

S. Lalondrelle
Royal Marsden Hospital, London, UK
e-mail: Susan.lalondrelle@rmh.nhs.uk

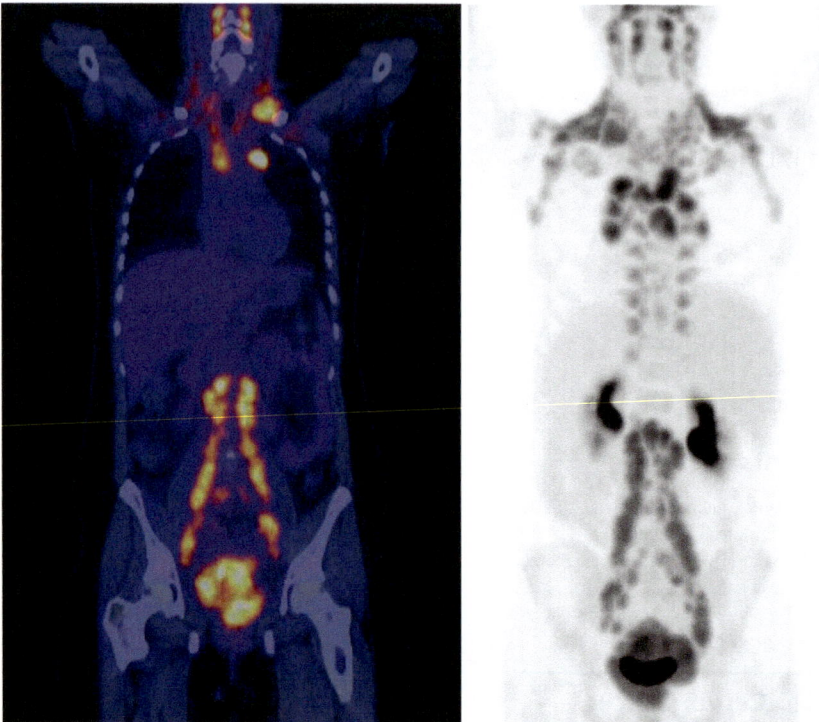

Fig. 12.1 Fused FDG-PET/CT for staging of cervical cancer demonstrating primary tumour and extensive lymphadenopathy extending from the pelvis to supraclavicular fossa

boost technique to simultaneously irradiate uninvolved lymph node chains. The nodal failure rate was <2%. Others have performed planning studies to model dose escalation up to 60 Gy whilst maintaining dose constraints to organs at risk [5, 6]. Clinical evidence for a dose response and optimal boost dose are however lacking.

Although MRI is established as the gold standard for brachytherapy planning, a few studies have assessed the use of PET. Malyapa et al. [7] reported the feasibility of performing PET with brachytherapy applicators in place. Lin et al. [8] compared PET-based dosimetry to the target volume with standard imaging and concluded that PET-based planning led to enhanced dose optimisation without increasing dose to organs at risk.

PET has also been studied to assess response during radiotherapy leading to adaptive planning based on functional volumes. Early lymph node complete response at 3 weeks can be correlated with an excellent prognosis [9] and local control [10]. These findings support the use of dose de-escalation in cases of initial good functional response, whilst poorly responding nodes and primary tumours can have plans adapted to escalate dose further.

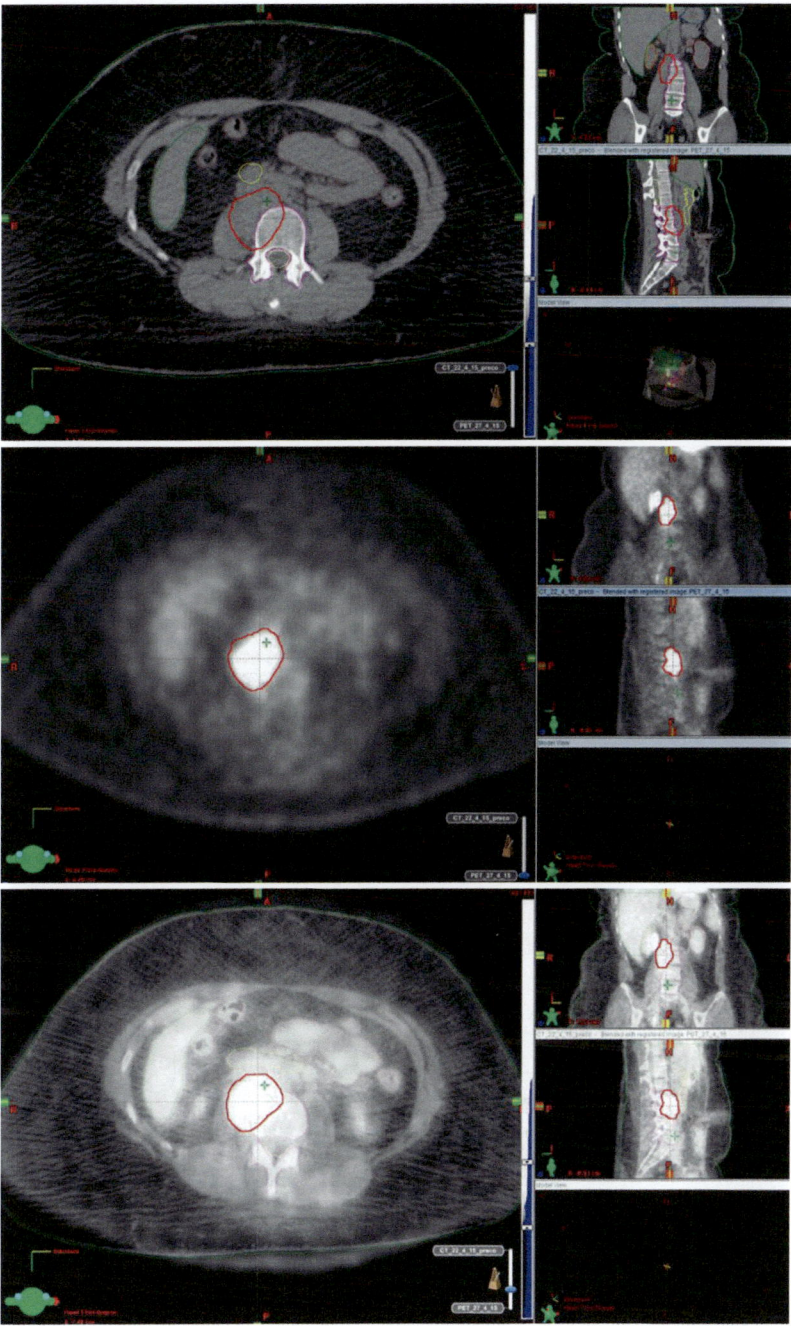

Fig. 12.2 Fusion of planning CT and PET to aid target delineation in a case of para-aortic nodal relapse. Non-contrast CT does not demonstrate the target well; fusion of PET imaging allows accurate depiction of target volume

12.2 Endometrial Cancer

The use of PET is less well established for endometrial cancer compared to cervical cancer. Its use lies mainly in the diagnosis of pelvic and distant metastatic disease, aiding decisions about pelvic lymph node dissection and in assessing local disease. As most radiotherapy delivered for endometrial cancer is delivered to the post-operative pelvis, no role for the use of PET in RT planning has yet been explored.

12.3 Novel PET Tracers

C-choline has the advantage of reduced urinary uptake, facilitating primary tumour identification in cervical cancer but with increased bowel uptake hampering nodal disease assessment. Comparison of ^{64}Cu-ATSM and ^{60}Cu-ATSM in cervix cancer found a better image quality with ^{64}Cu-ATSM, because of lower noise, and concluded that ^{64}Cu-ATSM appeared to be a safe radiopharmaceutical with high-quality images of tumour hypoxia. These hypoxic tracers may facilitate further clinical studies of functional dose painting in cervix cancer.

PET/CT is well established in the radiotherapy pathway for cervix cancer as a staging tool and for assessment of response. Increasingly it is incorporated into radiotherapy planning as a functional target for dose escalation.

> **Key Points**
> **Cervix Cancer**
>
> - ^{18}FDG PET/CT is routinely used in the staging of primary cervix cancer for assessment of nodal involvement and distant metastasis.
> - PET/CT has been incorporated into the radiotherapy planning process, primarily as an aid to defining nodal disease for dose escalation, but also for GTV definition.
> - PET/CT-based GTV delineation has been compared to MRI both to define the superior border of pelvic/para-aortic fields and in defining the primary target.
> - The main use of PET/CT in cervix radiotherapy planning has been the identification of lymph node targets for boosting dose. PET-based planning led to enhanced dose optimisation without increasing dose to organs at risk.
> - PET has also been studied to assess response during radiotherapy leading to adaptive planning based on functional volumes.
>
> **Endometrial Cancer**
>
> - Most radiotherapy delivered for endometrial cancer is delivered to the post-operative pelvis; no role for the use of PET in RT planning has yet been explored.

References

1. Narayan K, et al. A comparison of MRI and PET scanning in surgically staged loco-regionally advanced cervical cancer: potential impact on treatment. Int J Gynecol Cancer. 2001;11(4):263–71.
2. Upasani MN, et al. 18-fluoro-deoxy-glucose positron emission tomography with computed tomography-based gross tumor volume estimation and validation with magnetic resonance imaging for locally advanced cervical cancers. Int J Gynecol Cancer. 2012;22(6):1031–6.
3. Kidd EA, et al. Clinical outcomes of definitive intensity-modulated radiation therapy with fluorodeoxyglucose-positron emission tomography simulation in patients with locally advanced cervical cancer. Int J Radiat Oncol Biol Phys. 2010;77(4):1085–91.
4. Grigsby PW, et al. Lymph node control in cervical cancer. Int J Radiat Oncol Biol Phys. 2004;59:706–12.
5. Esthappan J, et al. Treatment planning guidelines regarding the use of CT/PET-guided IMRT for cervical carcinoma with positive paraaortic lymph nodes. Int J Radiat Oncol Biol Phys. 2004;58:1289–97.
6. Mutic S, et al. PET-guided IMRT for cervical carcinoma with positive para-aortic lymph nodes-a dose-escalation treatment planning study. Int J Radiat Oncol Biol Phys. 2003;55(1):28–35.
7. Malyapa RS, et al. Physiologic FDG-PET three-dimensional brachytherapy treatment planning for cervical cancer. Int J Radiat Oncol Biol Phys. 2002;54:1140–6.
8. Lin LL, et al. Adaptive brachytherapy treatment planning for cervical cancer using FDG-PET. Int J Radiat Oncol Biol Phys. 2007;67:91–6.
9. Bjurberg M, et al. Prediction of patient outcome with 2-deoxy-2-[18F]fluoro-D-glucose-positron emission tomography early during radiotherapy for locally advanced cervical cancer. Int J Gynecol Cancer. 2009;19(9):1600–5.
10. Yoon MS, et al. Metabolic response of pelvic and para-aortic lymph nodes during radiotherapy for carcinoma of the uterine cervix: using positron emission tomography/computed tomography. Int J Gynecol Cancer. 2011;21(4):699–705.

Paediatric Tumours

13

Lucy Fowkes and Sue Chua

Contents

13.1 Introduction 73
13.2 Indications 74
13.3 Patient Preparation 74
13.4 Scan Protocol 75
13.5 Tumour Delineation 75
References 76

13.1 Introduction

Radiotherapy (RT) is employed as a curative rather than palliative treatment in children with cancer. Paediatric cancers are rare, so use of positron emission tomography-computed tomography (PET/CT) to plan RT is typically performed by specialist centres. A physiologically heterogeneous population, ranging from neonate to adolescent, has practical implications for image acquisition, interpretation and RT dose. Increased susceptibility to the effects of ionising radiation leads to pronounced adverse effects, with the long-term risk of secondary malignancy amplified by concurrent chemotherapy and imaging studies performed during and after treatment [1].

L. Fowkes
Radiology & Radionuclide Radiology, The Royal Marsden NHS Foundation Trust, London, UK

S. Chua (✉)
Department of Nuclear Medicine and PET, Royal Marsden NHS Foundation Trust, Sutton, Surrey, UK
e-mail: sue.chua@rmh.nhs.uk

© Springer International Publishing Switzerland 2017
S. Chua (ed.), *PET/CT in Radiotherapy Planning*, Clinicians' Guides to Radionuclide Hybrid Imaging - PET/CT, DOI 10.1007/978-3-319-54744-2_13

Table 13.1 Evidence for PET/CT RT planning in children

Lesion	PET tracers	Evidence/use
Lymphoma	^{18}F-FDG	Most frequent indication for PET/CT RT planning [3]
		Facilitates involved nodal RT [4]
Wilm's tumour	^{18}F-FDG	Disease no longer confined to the kidney
Neuroblastoma	^{18}F-FDG	Not a widely used tracer in this tumour type but has shown some promise in poorly differentiated/123I-mIBG-negative neuroblastoma [5]
	^{18}F-DOPA	
	^{68}Ga DOTATATE	Highly sensitive and specific in the detection of neuroblastic tumours [6]
	^{124}I-mIBG	Clinical trial awaited
		Identifies disease potentially amenable to ^{177}Lu DOTATATE therapy [7]
		Ongoing research
		Predicts radiation doses from ^{131}I-MIBG [8]
Sarcoma	^{18}F-FDG	Improved disease detection alters treatment in rhabdomyosarcoma [9]
Brain	^{11}C-MET[a]	To delineate actual tumour volume
	^{18}F-FET[a]	To differentiate between true disease recurrence and pseudoprogression [10]
	^{18}F-FCH[a]	
	^{18}F-FLT	
	^{18}F-DOPA	

[a]Tracers mainly limited to research use but are increasingly being used in clinical practice
Where   *^{124}I-MIBG* ^{124}I-metaiodobenzylguanidine,   *^{68}Ga DOTATATE* ^{68}Ga 1,4,7,10-tetraazacyclotetradecane-*N*,*N′*,*N″*,*N‴*-tetraacetic acid-octreotate, *^{11}C-MET* ^{11}C-methionine, *^{18}F-FET* ^{18}F-fluoroethyl-l-tyrosine, *^{18}F-FCH* ^{18}F-choline, *^{18}F-FLT* ^{18}F-3′-deoxy-3′-fluorothymidine

Using PET/CT to plan RT can potentially reduce a child's radiation dose by clarifying areas of uncertainty on conventional imaging and aiding modification of RT dose in accordance with tumour metabolic response [2].

13.2 Indications

Experience using PET/CT tracers other than ^{18}F-fluorodeoxyglucose (^{18}F-FDG) in the paediatric population is limited although there are a number under study (Table 13.1).

13.3 Patient Preparation

It is important that both the child and their parents/guardians are adequately informed prior to the scan to ease any anxiety and aid compliance with the process. Any written and verbal information should be ideally provided before the appointment with an opportunity for parents to ask questions (Please also refer to Sect. 2.2: Patient Preparation and Set-up).

For RT planning this will necessitate an explanation and possible demonstration of the use of moulding foams and other immobilisation devices. The need for any premedication and/or anaesthesia should also be considered at this stage.

Premedication with a benzodiazepine [11] or propranolol [12] may be considered to suppress ^{18}F-FDG uptake by brown fat which may be a particular problem in older children [3], although controlling the patient's environmental temperature is an effective and preferable alternative [13].

Intravenous access should ideally be obtained prior to the patient's arrival to the nuclear medicine department to allay patient stress and increase procedural compliance. If there are difficulties achieving access, central venous catheters may be used, providing they are distant from suspected disease sites and adequately flushed with 0.9% normal saline after tracer injection [3].

13.4 Scan Protocol

Protocols for children should be designed with the focus upon reducing radiation dose; this is achieved by adjusting the amount of radiotracer injected according to the weight of the child (e.g. 3 MBq/kg for ^{18}F-FDG [3]) and CT tube current according to their size and imaging requirements. In the case of ^{18}F-FDG, tracer should be injected one hour before the PET scan. As is the procedure in adults, the patient should be kept warm; avoid exercise and talking during this period.

The table-top and fixation materials used for the PET/CT scan should be identical to those used in the accelerator to ensure reproducibility. Distraction with music or a video may help to minimise patient movement.

13.5 Tumour Delineation

On completion the scan is interpreted by a nuclear medicine physician/oncology radiologist, who determines the gross tumour volume (GTV-PET). Lesion contouring is then performed by visual analysis. The relevant volumes and images are then transferred to the RT dose planning system so treatment methods can be formulated.

> **Conclusion**
>
> Minimising irradiation of healthy tissue whilst maximising that delivered to the tumour target during RT is especially important in children, and PET/CT planning aids this process. With a continued need to improve treatment outcomes in this population, its application is set to increase.

Key Points

- Radiotherapy (RT) is employed as a curative rather than palliative treatment in children with cancer.

- Paediatric cancers are rare, so use of positron emission tomography-computed tomography (PET/CT) to plan RT is typically performed by specialist centres.

- Using PET/CT to plan RT can potentially reduce a child's radiation dose by clarifying areas of uncertainty on conventional imaging and aiding modification of RT dose in accordance with tumour metabolic response.

- Protocols for children should be designed with the focus upon reducing radiation dose.

- The table-top and fixation materials used for the PET/CT scan should be identical to those used in the accelerator to ensure reproducibility.

References

1. Meadows AT, et al. Second neoplasms in survivors of childhood cancer: findings from the Childhood Cancer Survivor Study cohort. J Clin Oncol. 2009;27(14):2356–62.
2. Krasin MJ, Hudson MM, Kaste SC. Positron emission tomography in pediatric radiation oncology: integration in the treatment-planning process. Pediatr Radiol. 2004;34(3):214–21.
3. Birk Christensen CB, Loft L, Kiil Berthelsen A. PET/CT radiotherapy planning in children. In: Kinggaard MH, Federspiel P, editors. PET/CT radiotherapy planning part 3: a technologist guide. Vienna: European Association of Nuclear Medicine; 2012. p. 67–71.
4. Maraldo MV, et al. The impact of involved node, involved field and mantle field radiotherapy on estimated radiation doses and risk of late effects for pediatric patients with Hodgkin lymphoma. Pediatr Blood Cancer. 2014;61(4):717–22.
5. Colavolpe C, et al. Utility of FDG-PET/CT in the follow-up of neuroblastoma which became MIBG-negative. Pediatr Blood Cancer. 2008;51(6):828–31.
6. Lu MY, et al. Characterization of neuroblastic tumors using 18F-FDOPA PET. J Nucl Med. 2013;54(1):42–9.
7. Gains JE, et al. 177Lu-DOTATATE molecular radiotherapy for childhood neuroblastoma. J Nucl Med. 2011;52(7):1041–7.
8. Seo Y, et al. Tumor dosimetry using [124I]m-iodobenzylguanidine microPET/CT for [131I] m-iodobenzylguanidine treatment of neuroblastoma in a murine xenograft model. Mol Imaging Biol. 2012;14(6):735–42.
9. Ricard F, et al. Additional Benefit of F-18 FDG PET/CT in the staging and follow-up of pediatric rhabdomyosarcoma. Clin Nucl Med. 2011;36(8):672–7.
10. Spehl TS, Gotz IS. PET/CT-based radiotherapy planning in brain malignancies. In: E.A.f.N. Medicine, editor. PET/CT radiotherapy planning part 3: a technologist guide. Vienna: European Association of Nuclear Medicine; 2012.
11. Rakheja R, et al. Intravenous administration of diazepam significantly reduces brown fat activity on 18F-FDG PET/CT. Am J Nucl Med Mol Imaging. 2011;1(1):29–35.
12. Gelfand MJ, et al. Pre-medication to block [(18)F]FDG uptake in the brown adipose tissue of pediatric and adolescent patients. Pediatr Radiol. 2005;35(10):984–90.
13. Garcia C, et al. Effective reduction of brown fat FDG uptake by controlling environmental temperature prior to PET scan: an expanded case series. Mol Imaging Biol. 2010;12(6):652–6.

Index

A
Acquisition and reconstruction
   CT
      diagnostic scanning, 24
      RT planning, deviation for, 24–25
   PET
      diagnostic scanning, 24
      RT planning, deviation for, 24
Active breathing control (ABC) method, 40
Adaptive radiotherapy, 53
Amplitude binning, 41
ARSAC guidelines, 24
Artefacts, 29
   metallic objects, 29
   non-malignant processes, 30
   in PET/CT, 29, 30
   potential sources, 31
   respiratory motion, 30, 31
   state-of-the-art PET/CT scanners, 29

B
Benzodiazepine, 75
BNMS guidelines, 24
Breath-hold techniques, 40

C
C-choline, 70
Cervix cancer, 67–69
Choline-PET/CT (C-PET/CT), 63–64
Clinical target volume (CTV), 4, 5, 52
^{64}Cu-ATSM, 34, 70

D
2-Deoxy-2-(^{18}F) fluoro-D-glucose, 23
Digital Imaging and Communications in Medicine (DICOM), 25

Disease delineation, 33, 34
Dominant intra-prostatic lesions (DIL), 64
Dose painting methods, 36, 53–54

E
Endometrial cancer, 70
Endoscopic ultrasound (EUS), 59, 60
External beam radiotherapy (EBRT), 3, 4

F
4D PET/CT, 40, 41, 46

G
GI malignancy, 57
   oesophageal and pancreatic cancer, 59–60
   rectal cancer, 57–58
Gross tumour volume (GTV), 4, 5, 52
Gynaecological cancers
   cervix cancer, 67–69
   endometrial cancer, 70
   novel PET tracers, 70

H
Head and neck cancers (HNC)
   dose painting and adaptive radiotherapy, 53
   FDG-PET/CT, strengths and weaknesses, 53
   staging, 51
   target volume definition, 52
   treatment response evaluation, 54
Hounsfield units (HUs), 15
Hypoxia, 47, 48

I
Instrumentation, 13–15
Intensity-modulated radiotherapy (IMRT), 34, 52–53
Intravenous access, 75

L
Lung cancer
　hypoxia, 47, 48
　maximum standardised uptake value, 45
　practical radiotherapy planning, 46–47
　primary bronchogenic carcinoma, treatment, 46–48

M
Magnetic resonance imaging (MRI), 4, 52, 58, 63, 64, 68

O
Oesophageal cancer, 59–60
Oligometastatic disease, 64
Organs at risks (OARs), 5, 13

P
PACS systems, 25
Paediatric tumours, 73
　indications, 74
　patient preparation, 74–75
　scan protocol, 75
　tumour delineation, 75
Pancreatic cancer, 59–60
PET/CT
　advantages
　　disease delineation, accuracy in, individualizing radiotherapy treatment, 33–34
　limitations, 35–36
　RT planning, 4–8
　　artefacts, 29–31
　　data acquisition, reconstruction and transfer, 23–25
　　GI malignancy, 57–60
　　gynaecological cancers, 67–70
　　HNC, 51–54
　　instrumentation, 13–15
　　lung cancer, 45–48
　　paediatric tumours, 73–75
　　patient preparation, 17–21
　　prostate cancer, 63–64
PET-MRI, 7–8
Phase binning, 40
Propranolol, 75
Prostate cancer
　target volume delineation, 64
　treatment, patient selection, 63–64

R
Radiotherapy (RT) planning
　PET/CT, 4–7, 13–15
　　artefacts, 29–31
　　data acquisition, reconstruction and transfer, 23–25
　　GI malignancy, 57–60
　　gynaecological cancers, 67–70
　　HNC, 51–54
　　instrumentation, 13–15
　　lung cancer, 45–48
　　paediatric tumours, 73–75
　　patient preparation, 17–21
　　prostate cancer, 63–64
　target volumes in, 4
Reconstruction. *See* Acquisition and reconstruction
Rectal cancer, 57–58
Respiratory gating, 25
Respiratory motion, 30, 31, 39
RT planning. *See* Radiotherapy (RT) planning

S
SNM guidelines, 24
Specific uptake value (SUV), 36

T
Treatment planning systems (TPSs), 15
Tumour delineation, 75

GPSR Compliance

The European Union's (EU) General Product Safety Regulation (GPSR) is a set of rules that requires consumer products to be safe and our obligations to ensure this.

If you have any concerns about our products, you can contact us on ProductSafety@springernature.com

In case Publisher is established outside the EU, the EU authorized representative is:

Springer Nature Customer Service Center GmbH
Europaplatz 3
69115 Heidelberg, Germany

Batch number: 09745537

Printed by Printforce, the Netherlands